I'm No Quack

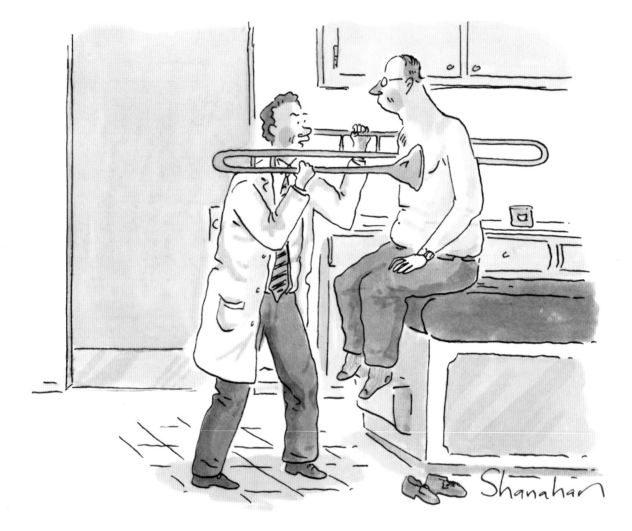

"Any family history of ragtime?"

I'm No Quack

A Book of Doctor Cartoons

by Danny Shanahan

Harry N. Abrams, Inc., Publishers

A C K N O W L E D G M E N T S

Thanks to everyone at the New Yorker, *the Cartoon Bank, and Abrams Books,*
and to all of the doctors whose combined efforts have managed to keep
me (reasonably) sane and healthy.

Project Manager: Christopher Sweet
Editor: Isa Loundon
Designer: Robert McKee
Production Manager: Maria Pia Gramaglia

Library of Congress Cataloging-in-Publication Data

Shanahan, Danny.
 I'm no quack! : a book of doctor cartoons /
by Danny Shanahan.
    p. cm.
 Includes bibliographical references and index.
 ISBN 0–8109–5799–X (hardcover : alk. paper)
1. Physicians—Caricatures and cartoons.
2. American wit and humor, Pictorial. I. Title.

NC1429.S49A4 2005a
741.5'973—dc22
                              2004030410

Printed and bound in China

10 9 8 7 6 5 4 3 2 1

ABRAMS

Harry N. Abrams, Inc.
100 Fifth Avenue
New York, N.Y. 10011
www.abramsbooks.com

Abrams is a subsidiary of

LA MARTINIÈRE
GROUPE

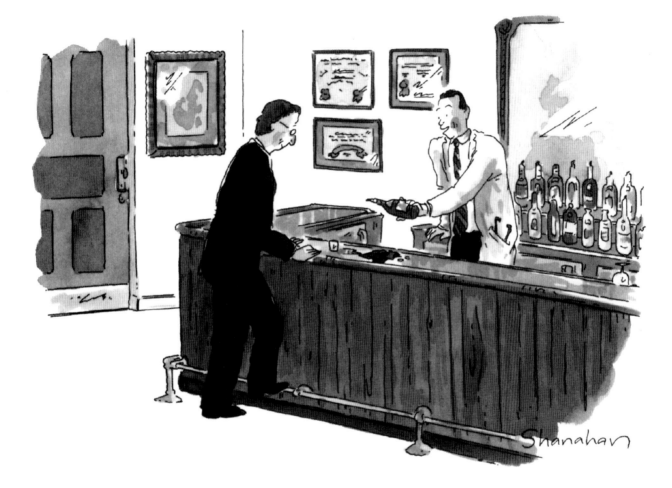

"And one for the old prostate."

To Dr. David Lemon (and his wonderful family), and in loving memory of Dr. Paul Branca and Dr. Al Stetson.

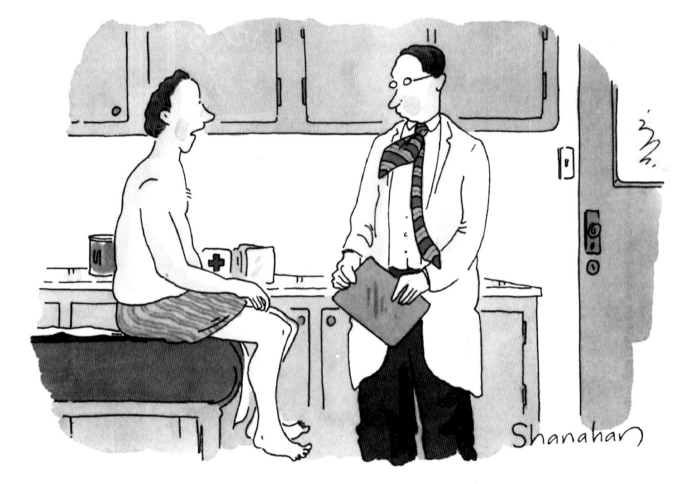

"And would you be performing the actual surgery?"

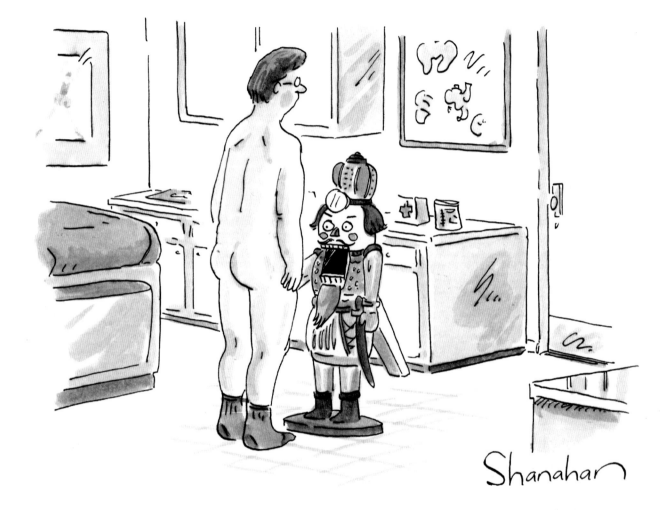

"Turn your head and scream."

Shanahan

Introduction

"Heel thyself."
—*Hippocrates's dog*

So, let's see if I've got this straight: scissors beats paper; rock beats scissors; paper beats rock. Every child knows that. Of course, as adults we know that in the hands of a trained physician a pair of scissors doesn't stand a chance of competing with a more-than-razor-sharp scalpel, not to mention the hewing and rending ability of a surgical laser. A rock? Granted, we've been bashing each other over the head with those babies for centuries, but, seriously, a rock? Any anesthesiologist worth his or her salt would bust a gut. Sure, a brick to the head will put even the feistiest patient under, but ever since ether, and up through morphine, codeine, and Demerol, they've been inventing new and exciting ways (if only slightly less harmful and invasive) to administer an M.D. T.K.O. Last, but not least, nobody does paper like the medical profession. Paper, when wielded by a doctor (and said doctor's loyal staff), trumps everything. The clipboard and pen (with that annoying little chain) may play their part, but it's the infernal, overwhelming, never-ending, repetitive, repetitive, repetitive, paperwork, paperwork, paperwork that kicks our shins, musses our hair, and beats us into the ground. If you're having trouble following me, if you haven't quite caught my drift, let me state it in the clearest possible way:

Doctors rule the world.

Yes, Virginia, it's true. Under the mild-mannered, care-giving, do-no-harm façade of even the humblest, most likeable small-town pediatrician lurk the despotic, megalomaniacal, do-as-I-say-not-as-I-do urges that, at any time, at the slightest whim or provocation, can bubble to the surface, scaring the suckers right out of the mouths of both innocent, vaccinatable toddlers and honest, hardworking lollipop lovers like you and I.

So, what to do? Do we let doctors push us around, meekly taking our medicine, rolling over and gritting our teeth, assuming the stirruped position, turning our heads and coughing, all without a fight, without the slightest bit of defiance? Or do we take a stand and hit them where it hurts?

I don't know about the rest of you, but this book is my stand, a first salvo in the battle, a comedic broadside aimed at those high-handed healers who, granted, may be saving tens of thousands of lives a year, and who, I suppose, could one day come up with one of those cancer cures or AIDS vaccines, and who, okay, give out a lot of cool little sample packets of the latest healing breakthroughs, both Marvin Gaye–type and non–Marvin Gaye–type— not that I'd be caught dead using the Marvin Gaye–type stuff, never even tried it, don't want it, don't need it—but who still need to be taken down a notch or two, or three! And I'm just the cartoonist to do it! And I'd like you DOCTORS to try and STOP ME!!!

Phew…my heart. I feel faint. Enjoy the book; I need to take my medication.

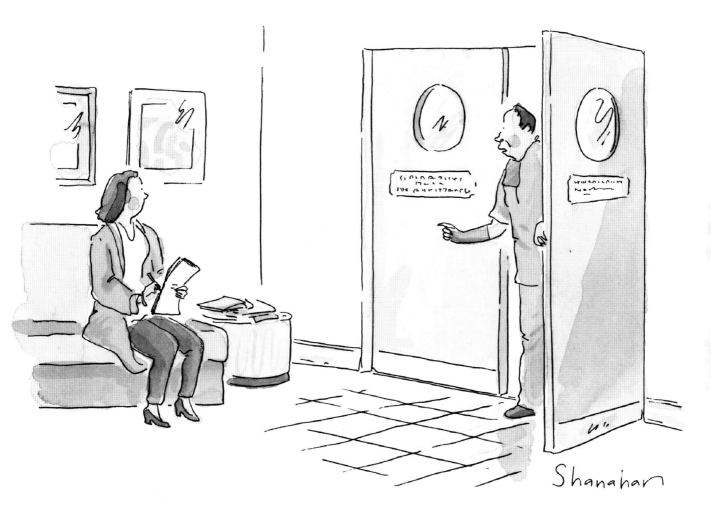

"Good news—a four-letter word for 'earthen pot' is 'olla.'"

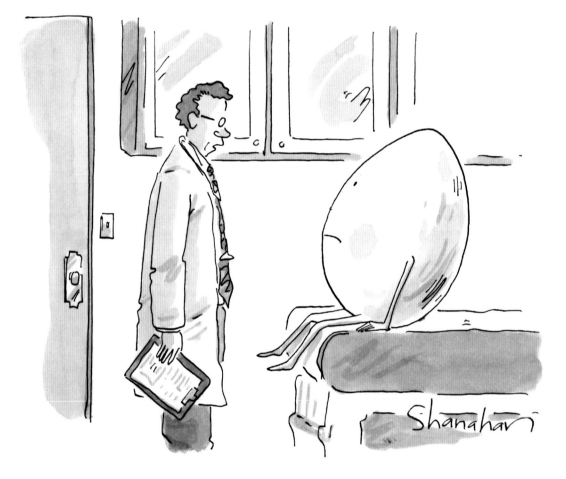

"We found a lumpty."

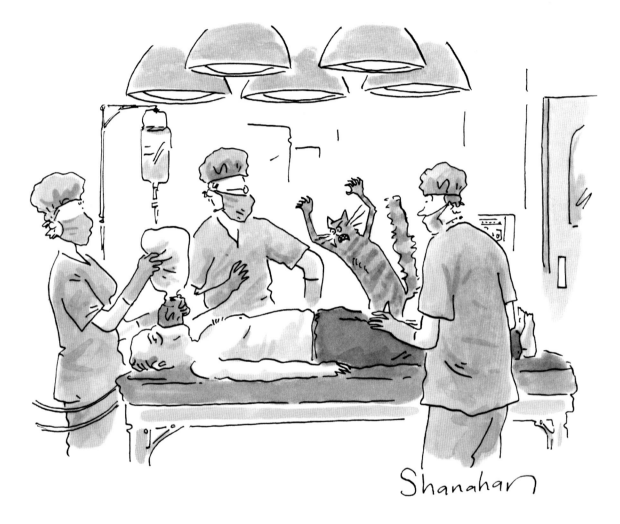

"CLEAR!"

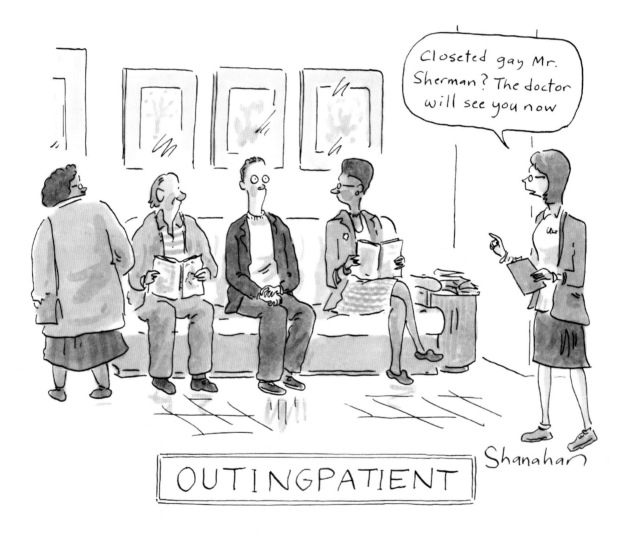

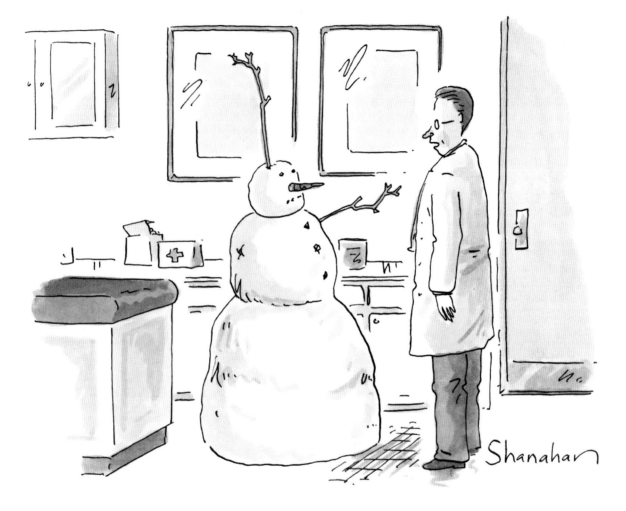

"It's dislocated, alright."

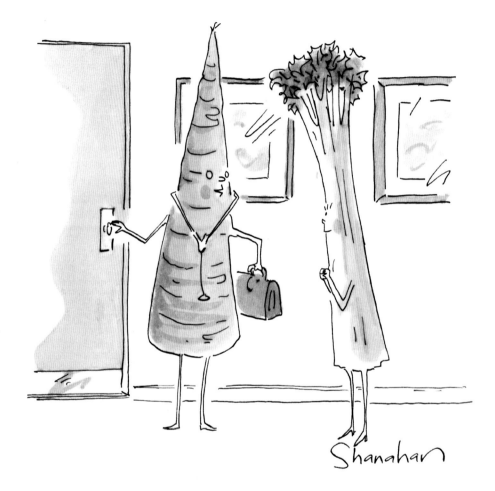

"He's doing great—he'll be back in a vegetative state in no time."

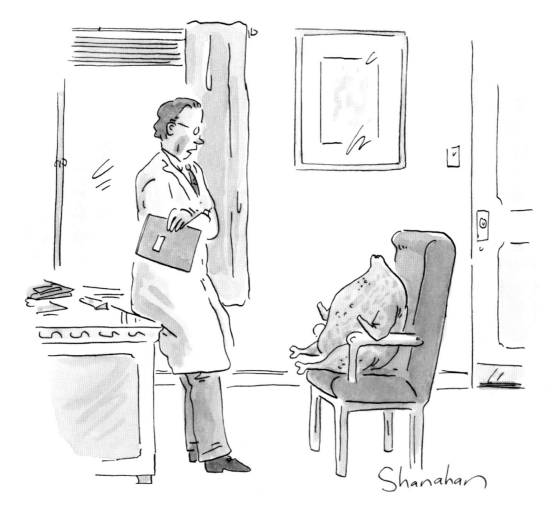

"*Your entire body is riddled with chestnuts.*"

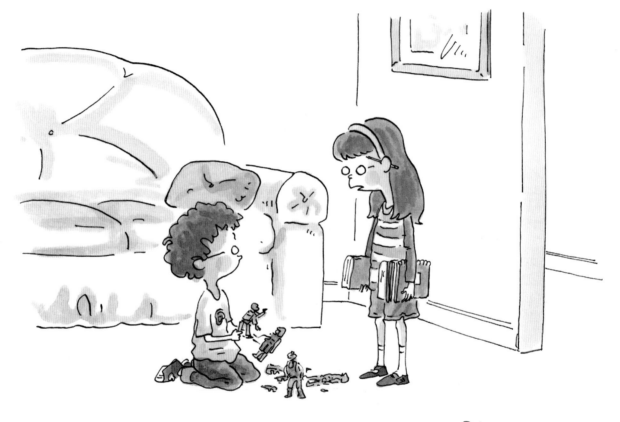

"Do you want to play doctorate?"

Shanahan

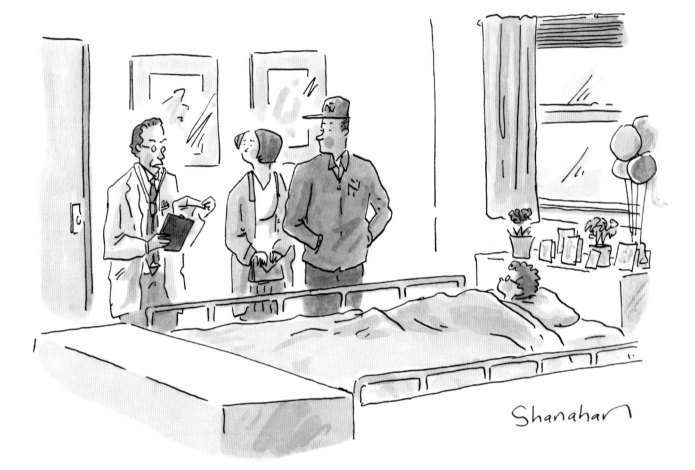

"*I'm sorry, Timmy, but Mr. Jeter's promise to hit you a home run isn't covered by your existing HMO.*"

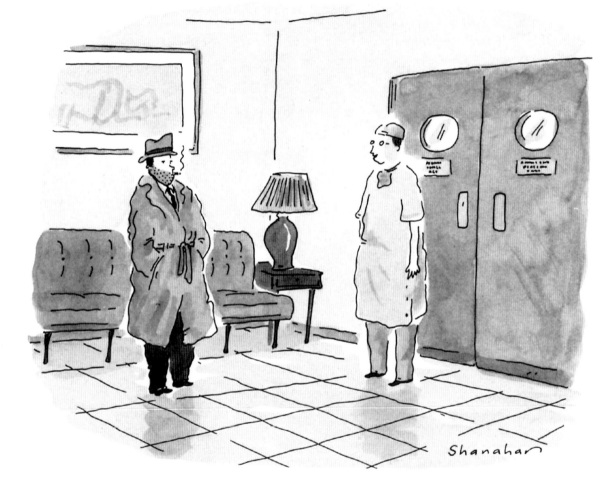

"It's a dame!"

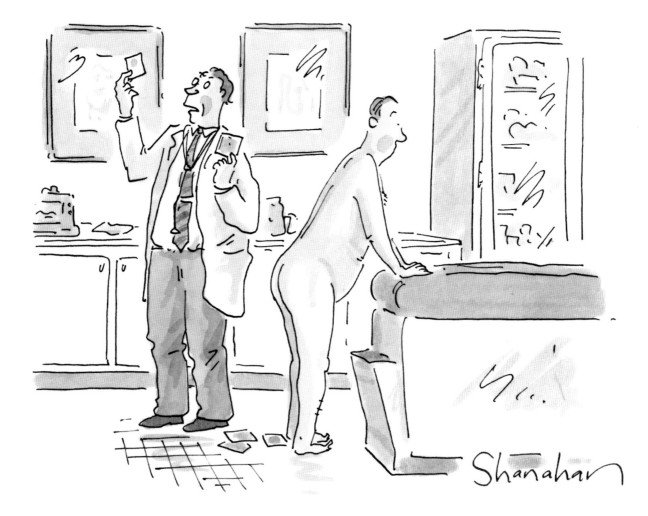

"*You have Polaroids.*"

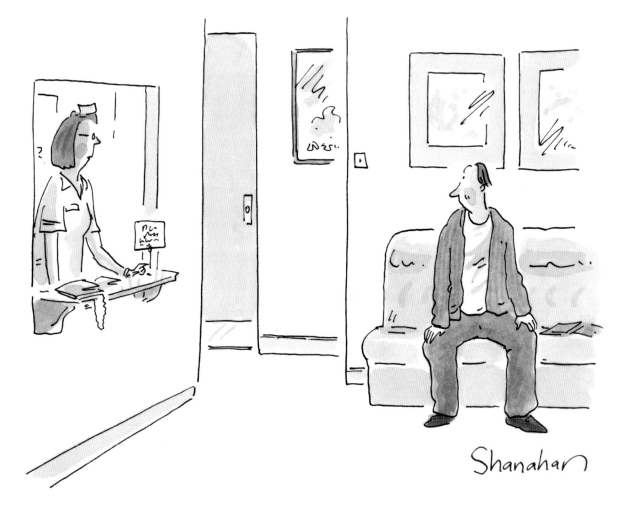

"Our medical intuitive will read you now."

Shanahan

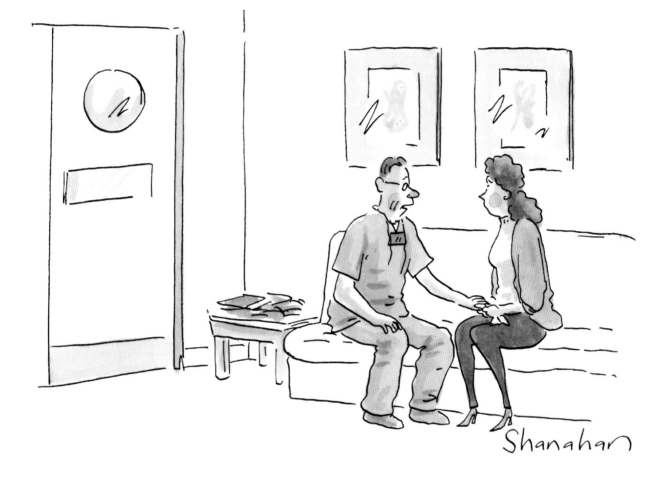

"His insides were all slimy and disgusting, but I'm told that's normal."

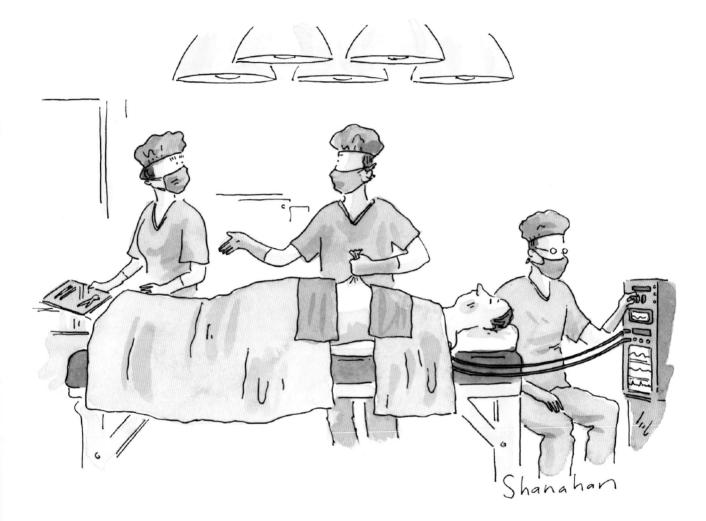

"Scrunchy."

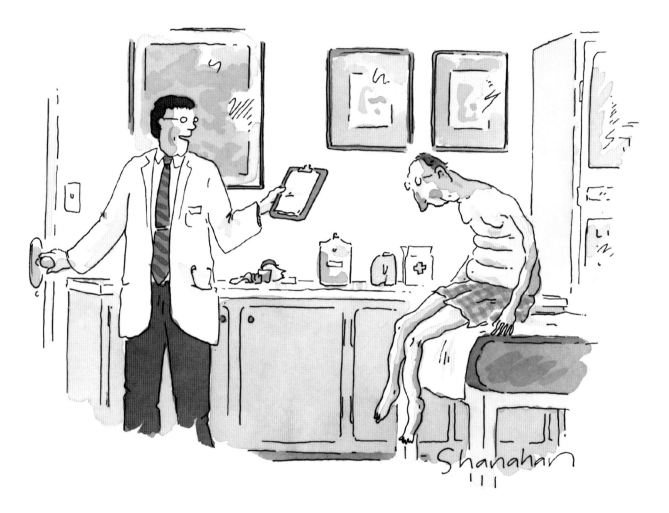

"Good news, Mr. Pickett—it's just a slow leak."

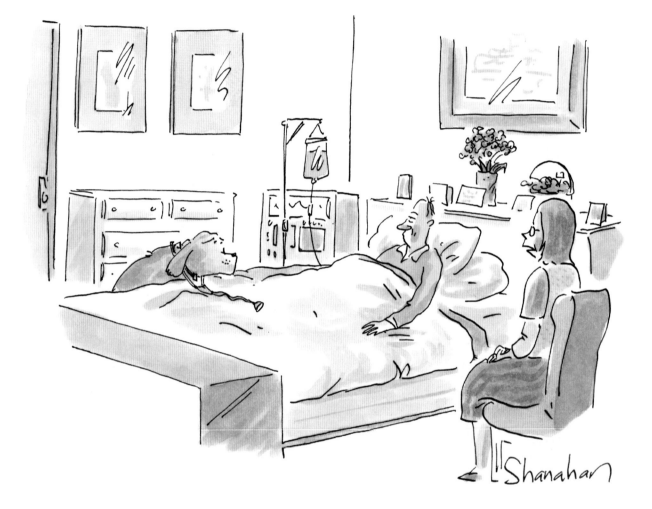

"On the other hand, his bedside manner is impeccable."

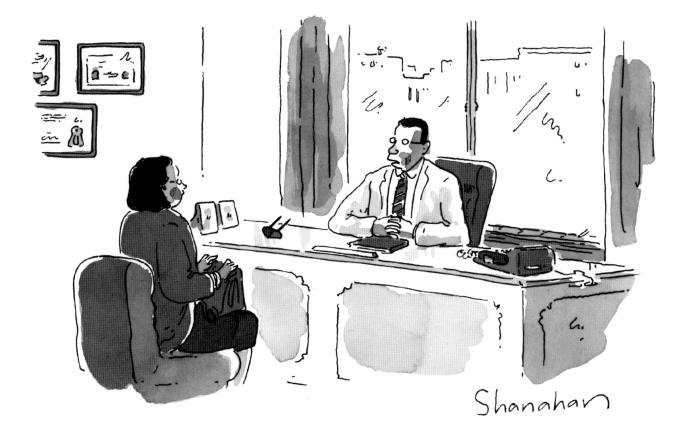

"You can rest assured, Mrs. Wilson, that your husband will receive the best care known to medical coverage."

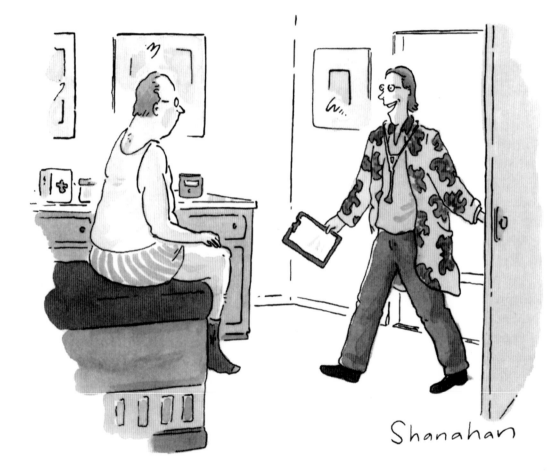

"So, let's catch a wellness wave!"

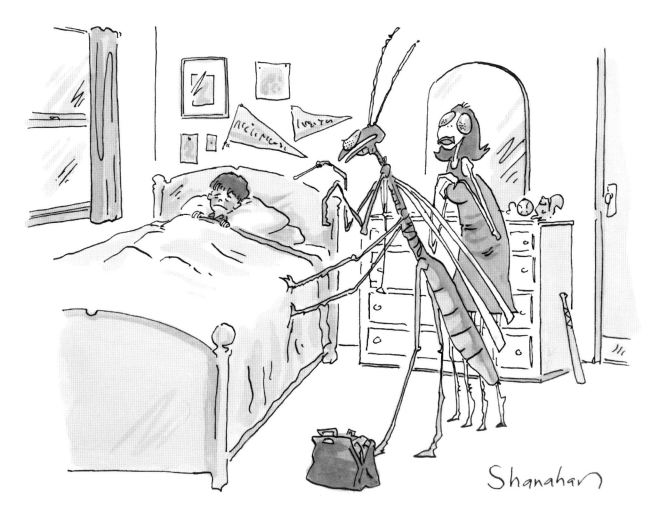

"He has a fevered imagination."

Shanahan

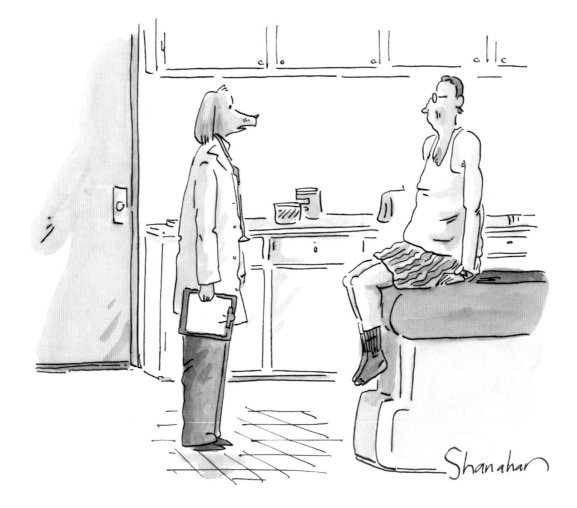

"Eat grass 'til you puke, then call me in the morning."

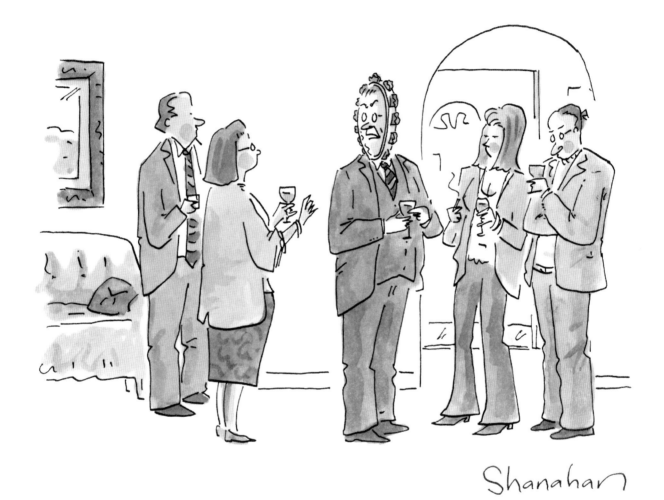

"*That's* Doctor *Tambourine Man.*"

Shanahan

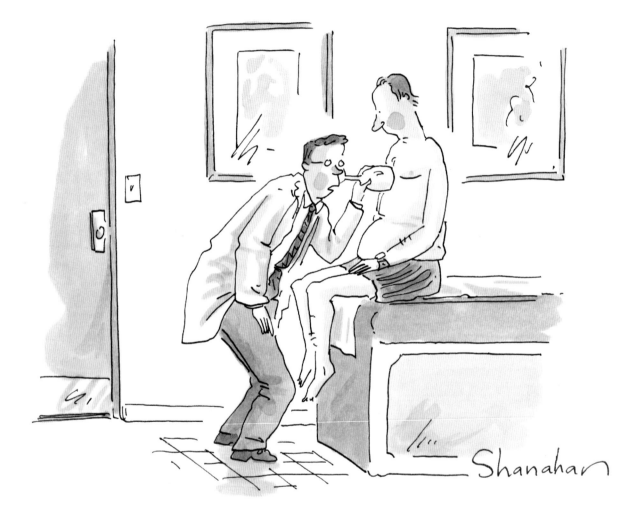

"Persistent, well-rounded, and full-bodied, with hints of smoke, and just a soupçon of irregularity."

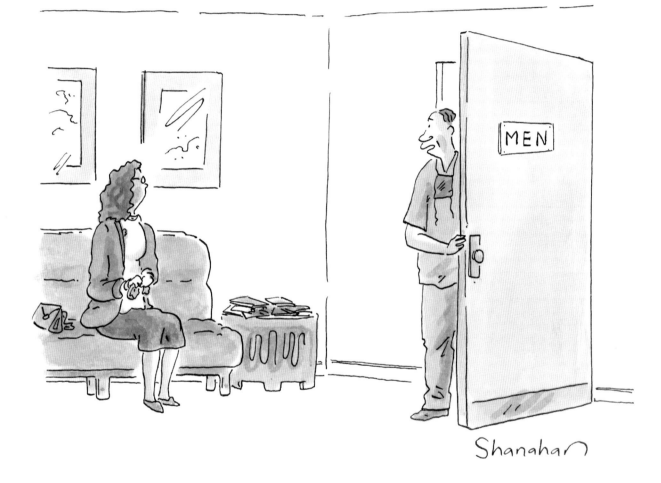

"We're doing all we can, Mrs. Fox, but he's already lost a lot of urine."

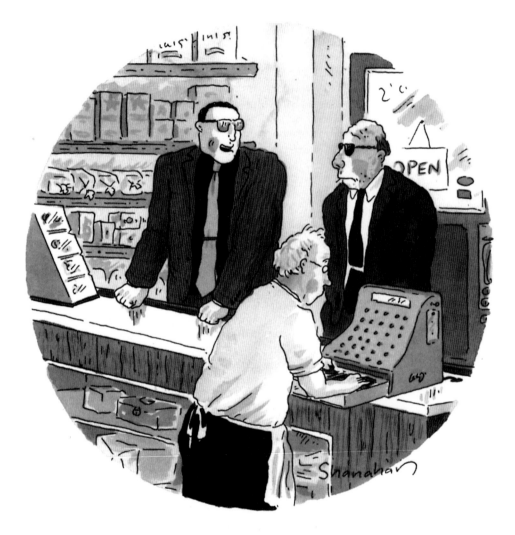

"Protection is a thing of the past, Eddie. You're looking at a supplemental-health-care provider."

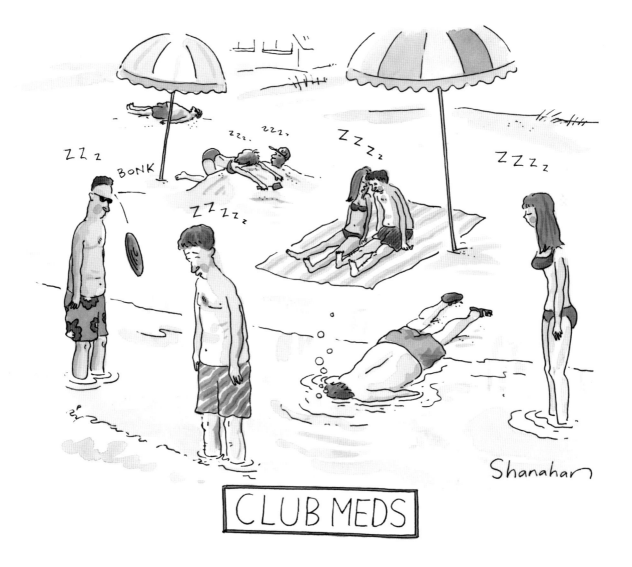

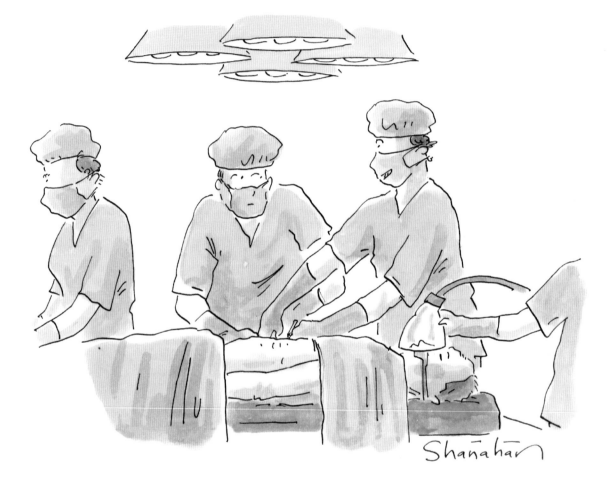

"Pull my finger."

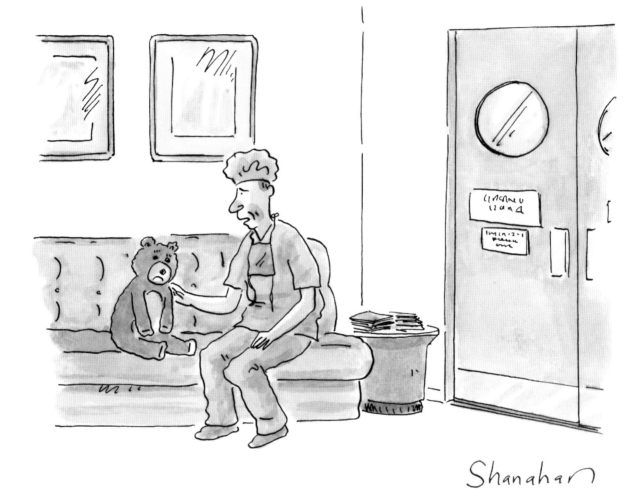

"We're pretty sure it was the dissolving stitches."

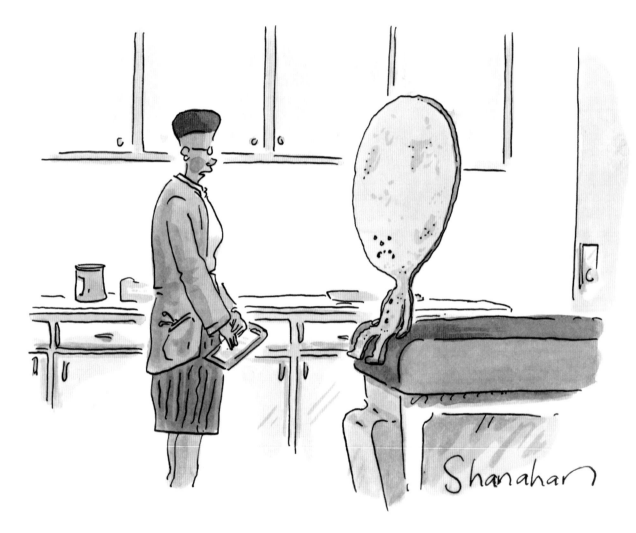

"You have a yeast infection."

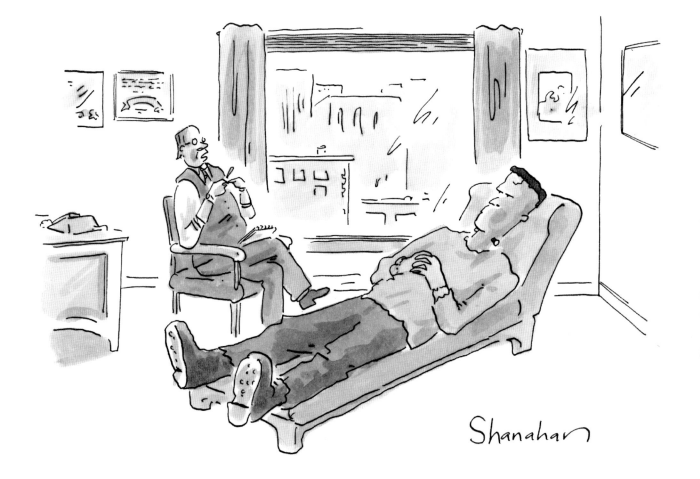

"*Tell me more about the voices in your neck.*"

Shanahan

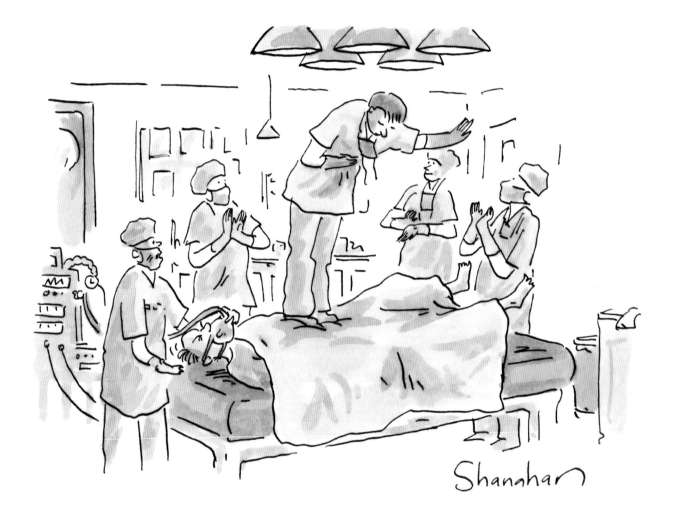

"He's coming out of it, Doc. Last encore."

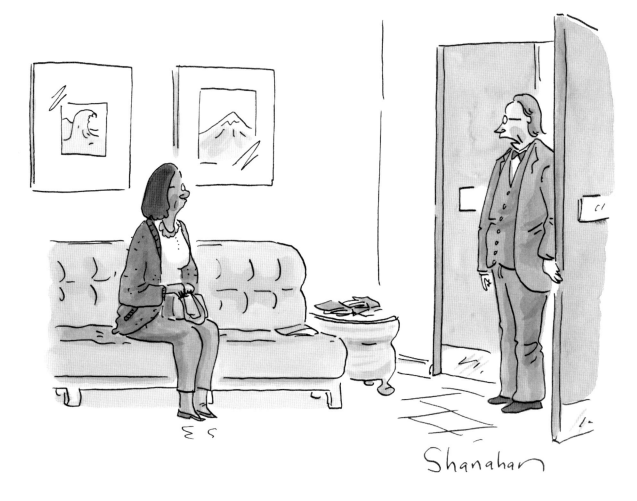

"He's gonna need more than a PhD."

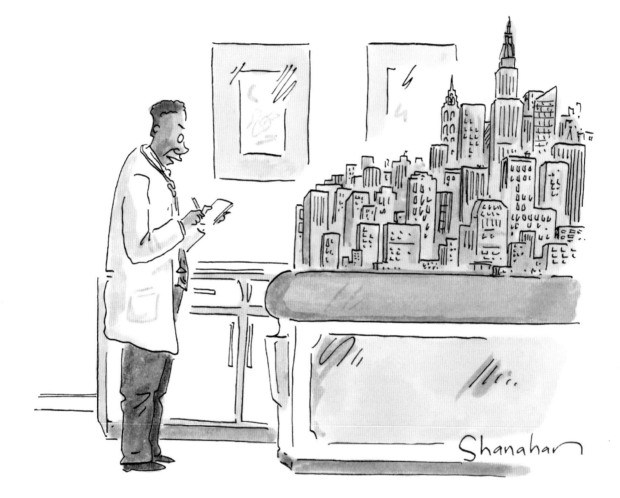

"*I'm going to give you something to help you sleep.*"

Shanahan

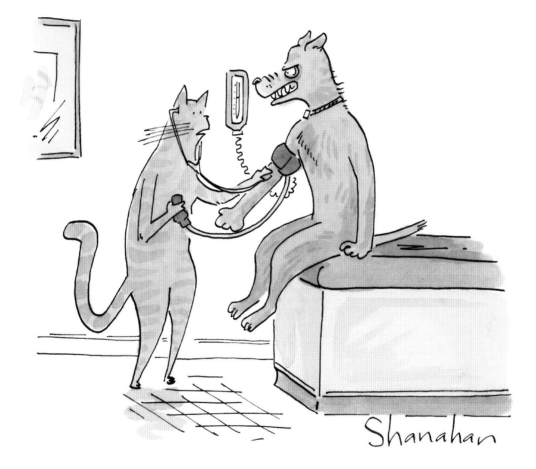

"Hm, still sky high. Let's try the other arm."

Shanahan

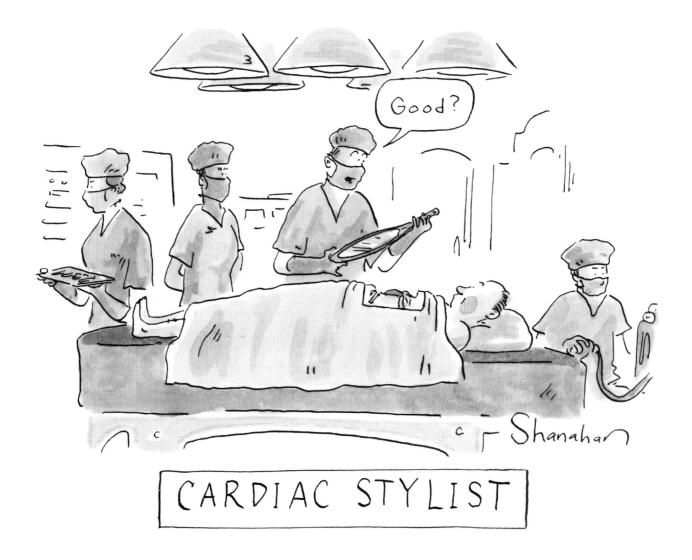

CARDIAC STYLIST

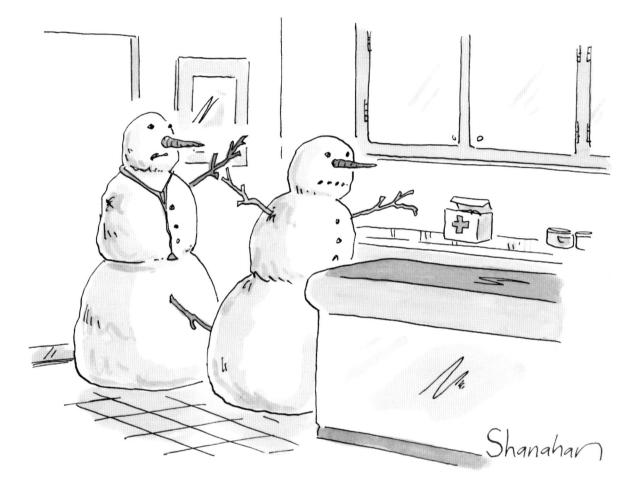

"Your prostate is enlarged."

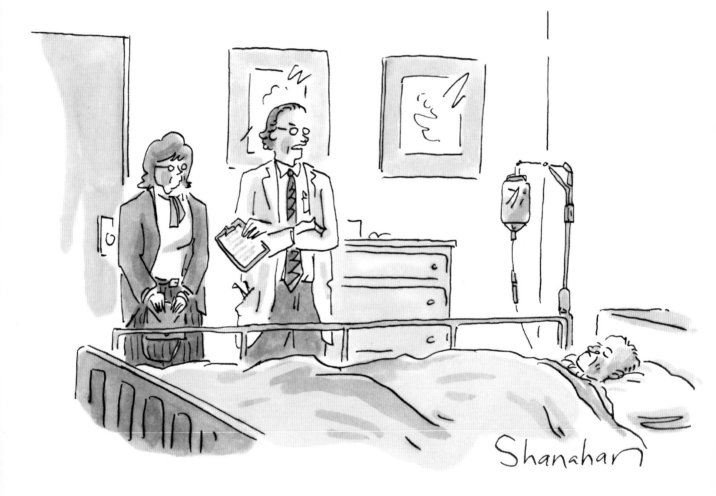

"No can do, Mrs. DePetrio. I'd be breaking my watchamacallit oath."

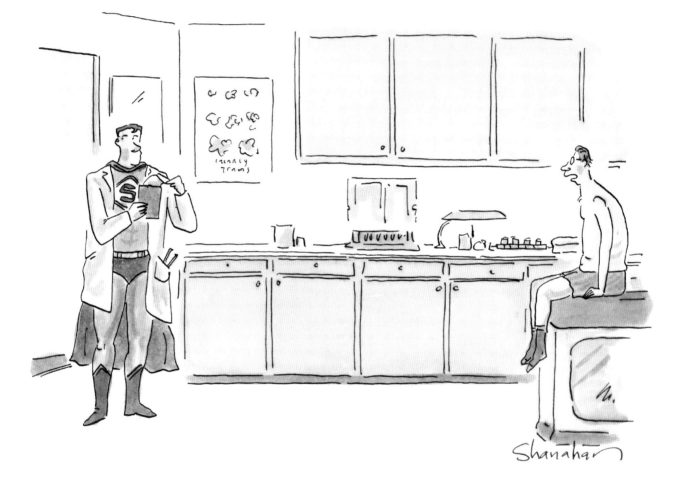

"If it's such a simple procedure, why can't we remove the kryptonite right here and now?"

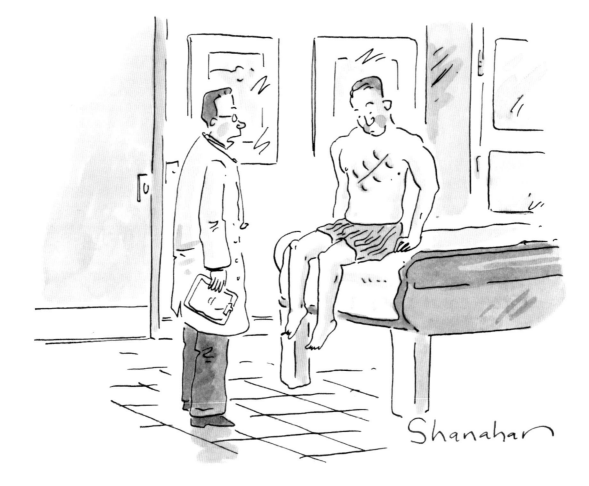

"They're washboard abs, Mr. Hunzinger, and they're on the move."

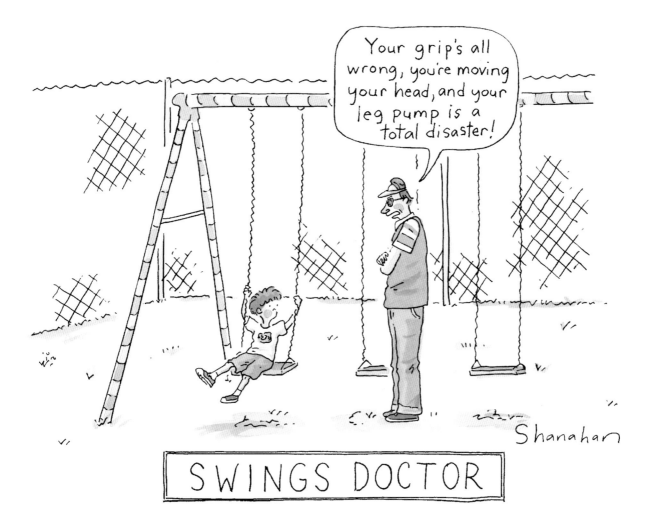

SWINGS DOCTOR

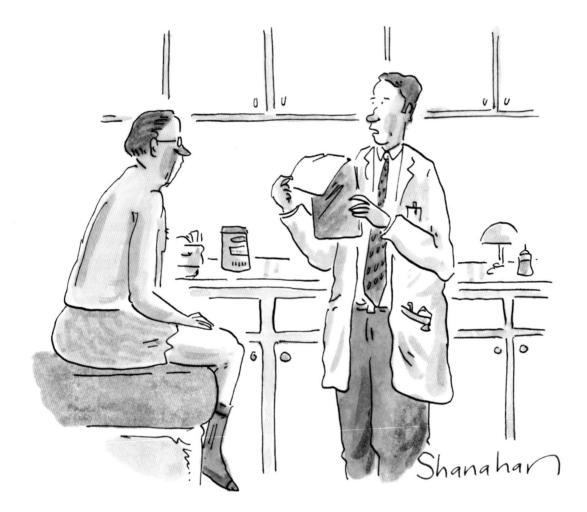

"Your condition's not rare, but it's very, very collectible."

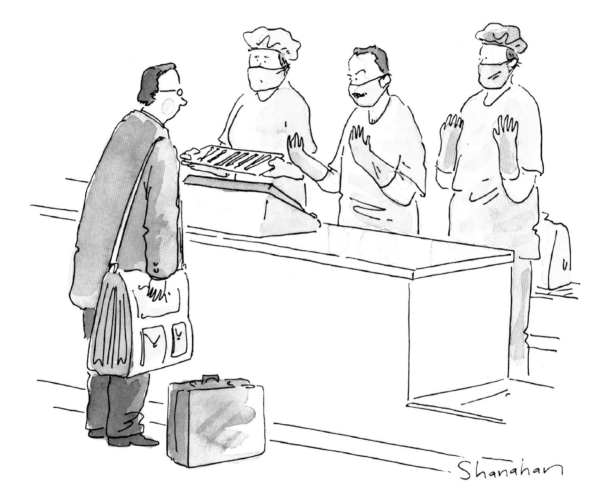

"I can get you to San Francisco through Dallas via Atlanta, but we'd have to take a kidney out right here and now."

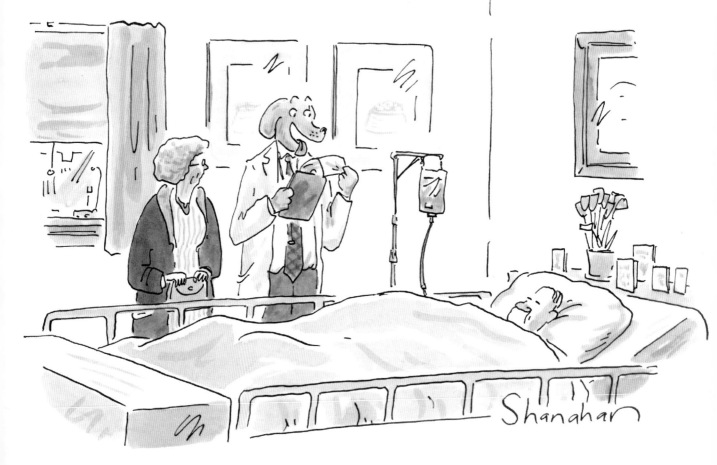

"*You can never run too many bone marrow tests.*"

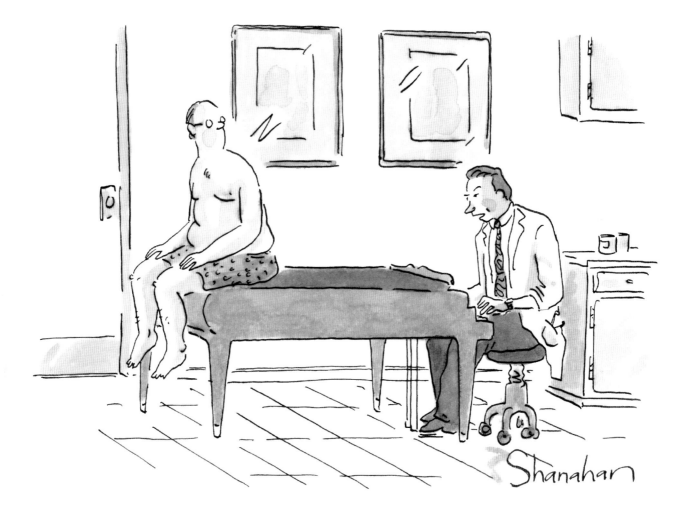

"Lemme tell you how I feel about high blood pressure, Mr. McGuinn."

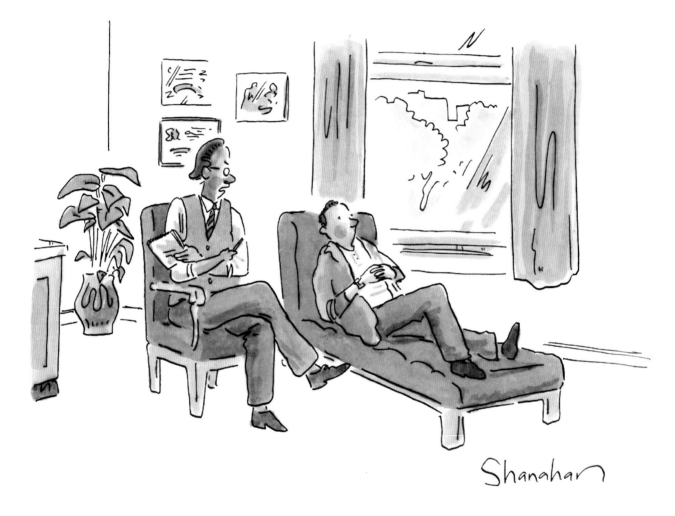

"*My, aren't we patient-oriented this morning.*"

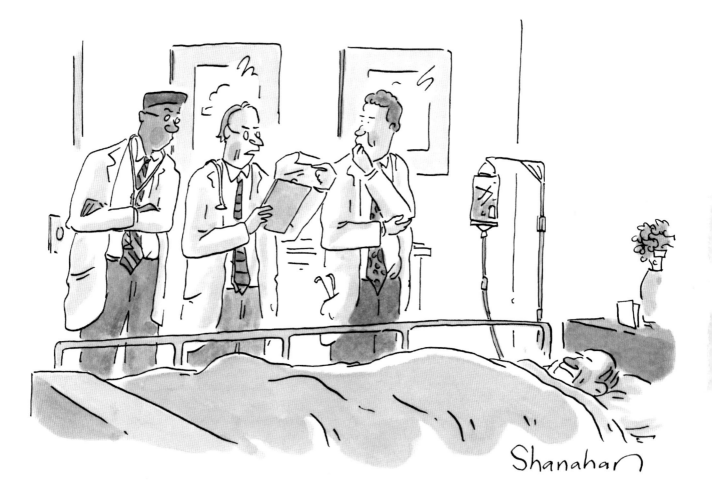

"By the time we got him in here, he had already lost an awful lot of liquidity."

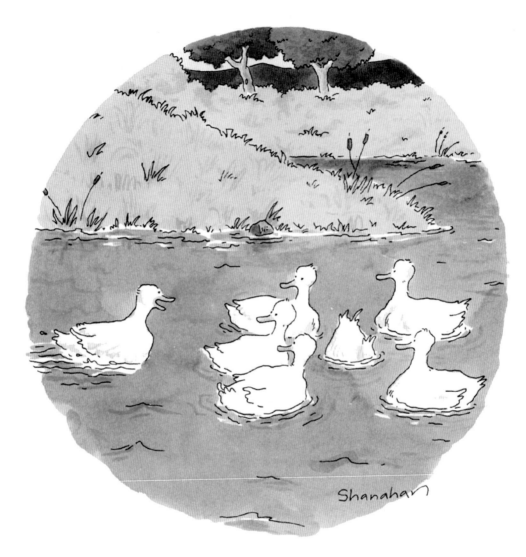

"Let me through! I'm a quack."

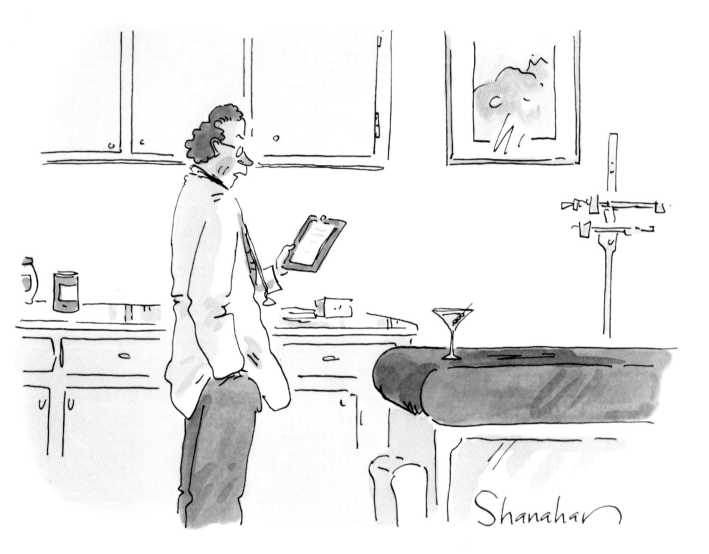

"You're painfully dry?"

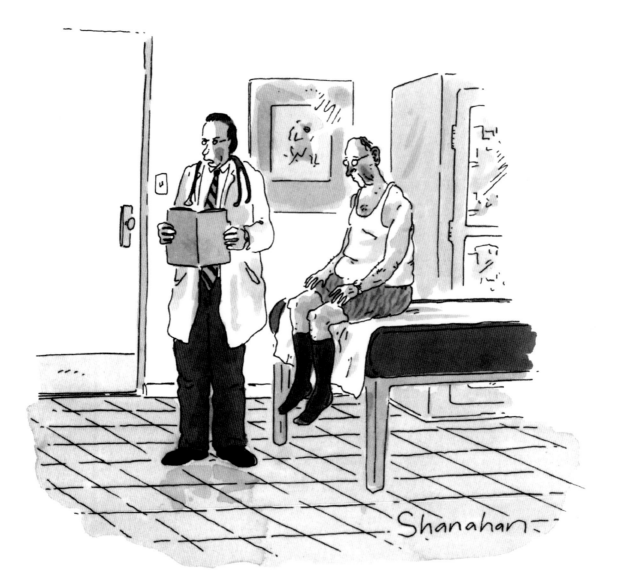

"Trust me, senator. Many people have active and fulfilling sex lives long after they've retired from Congress."

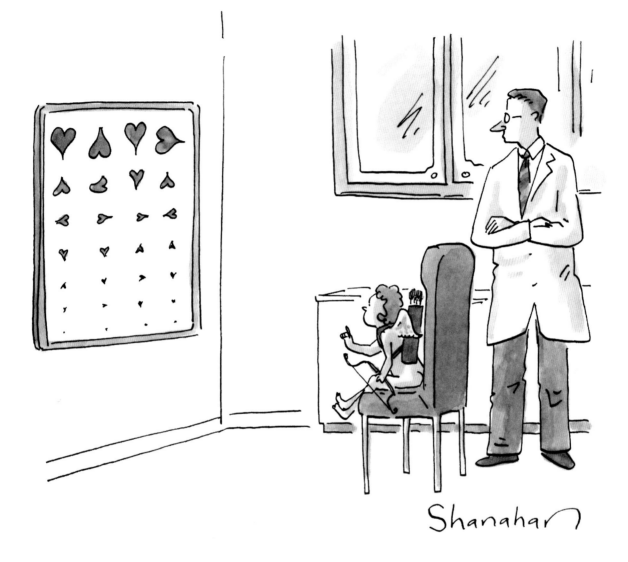

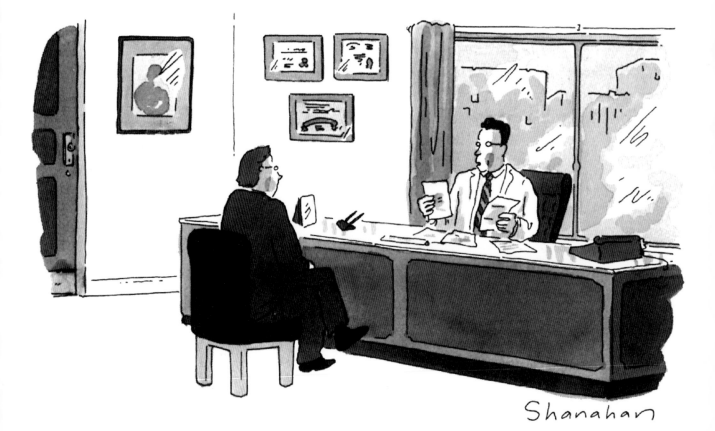

"You're responding beautifully. Let's go ahead and see what happens if we increase your deductible."

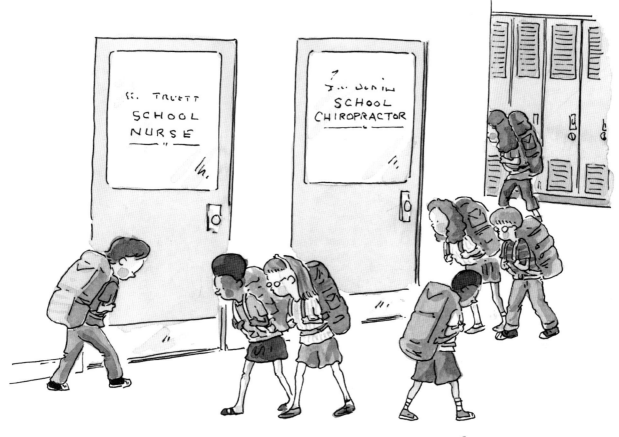

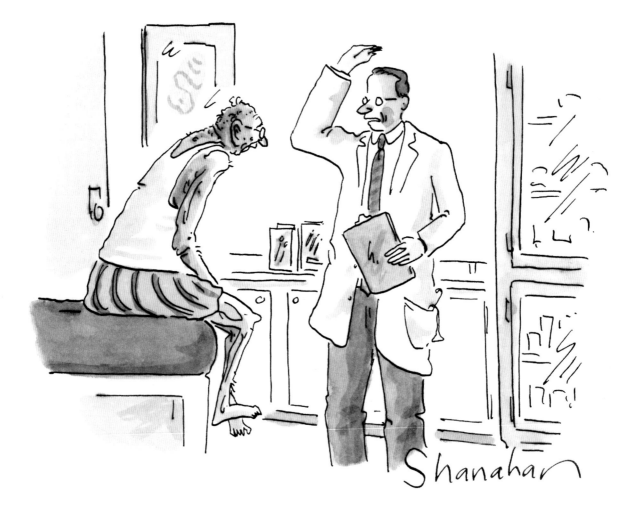

"I'm sorry, but you've had it up to here."

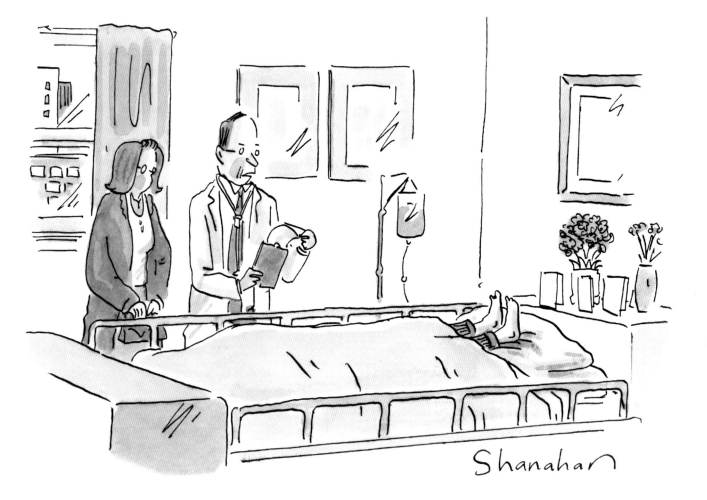

"He seems to have done a complete turnaround."

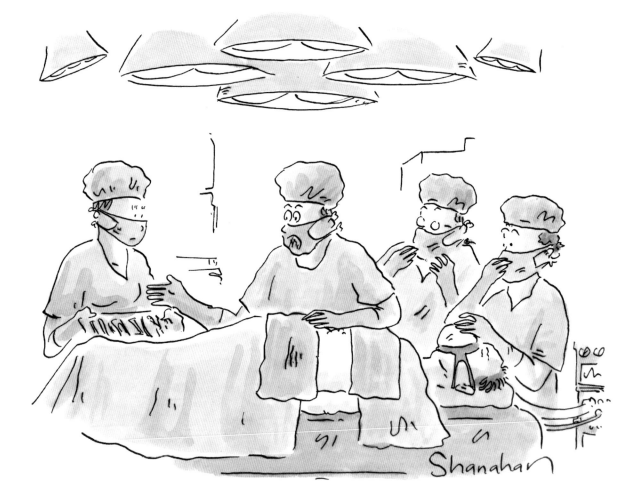

"Magic wand, stat!"

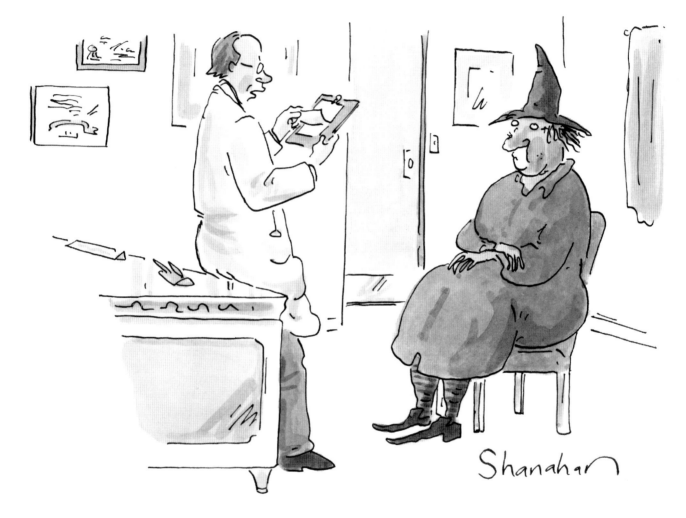

"Your next fattened child could be your last."

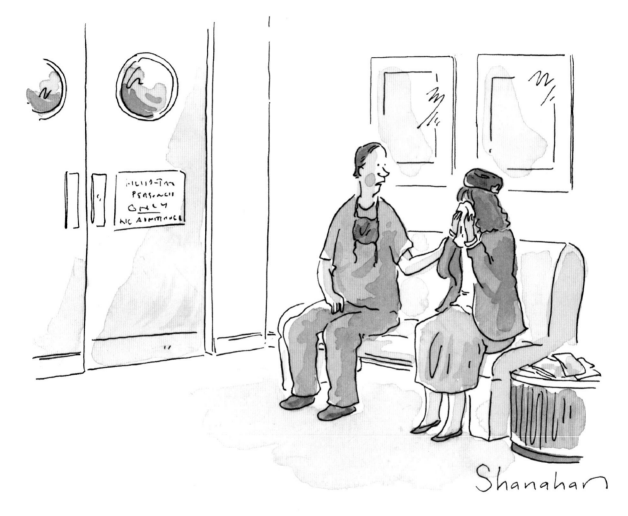

"His underwear was spotless."

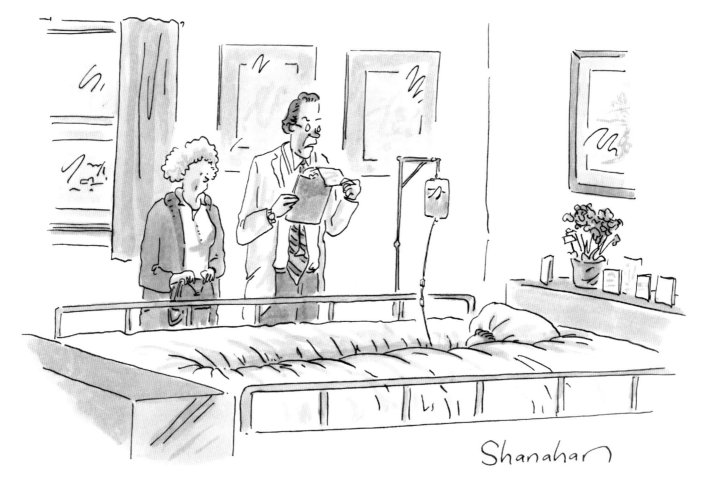

"Bone density looks good."

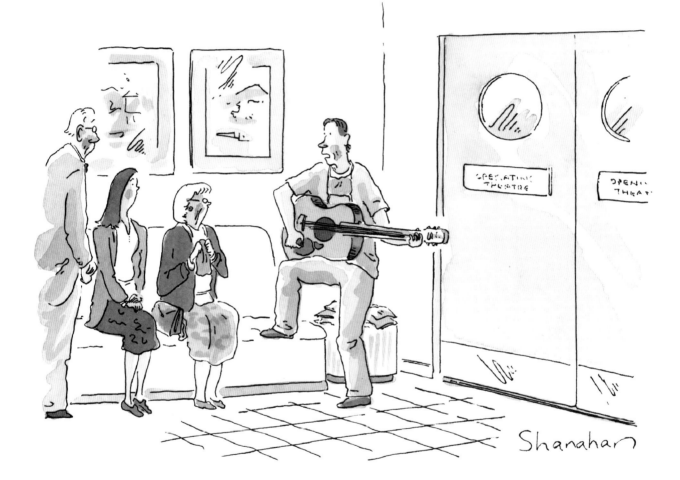

"Listen up, my fine people, and I'll sing you song, 'bout a brave neurosurgeon who done something wrong."

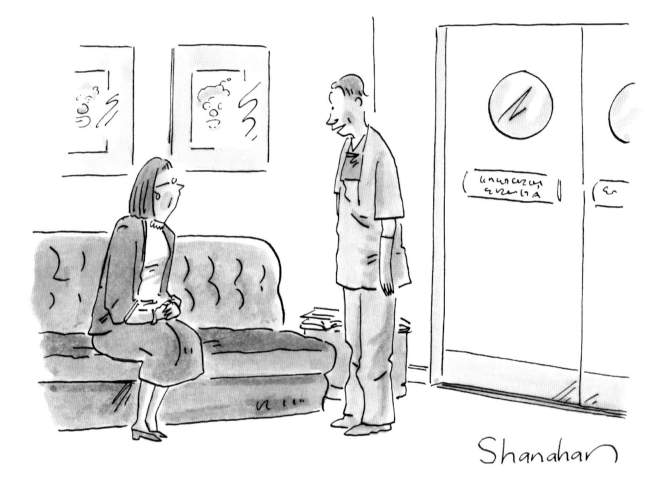

"There was a system failure that caused a brief crash, but fortunately I was able to reboot."

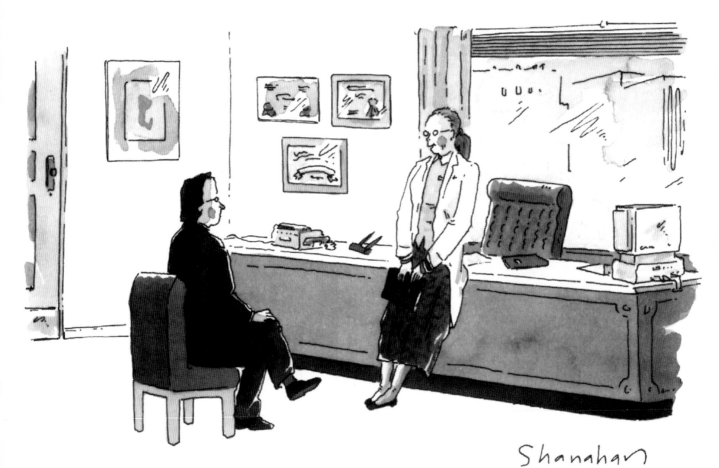

"Our integrated approach to medicine skillfully combines an array of holistic alternative treatments with a sophisticated computerized billing service."

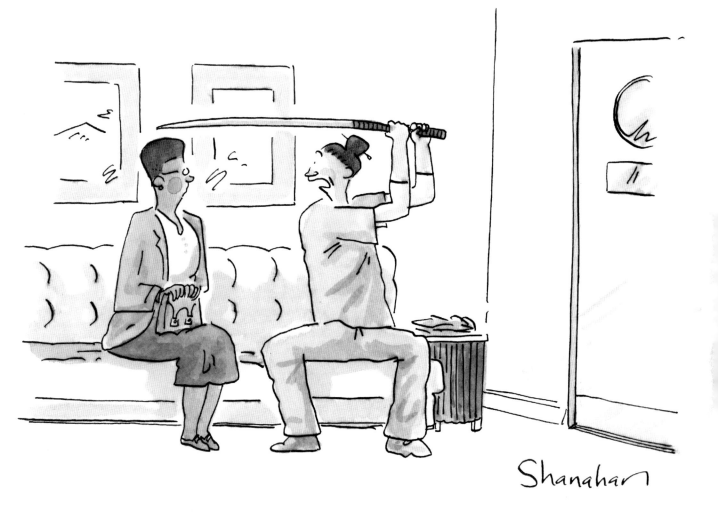

"There might be some scarring."

Shanahan

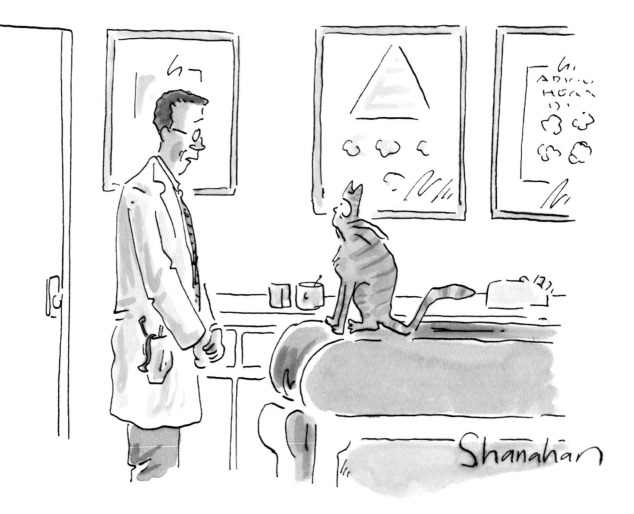

"*It's mouseborne.*"

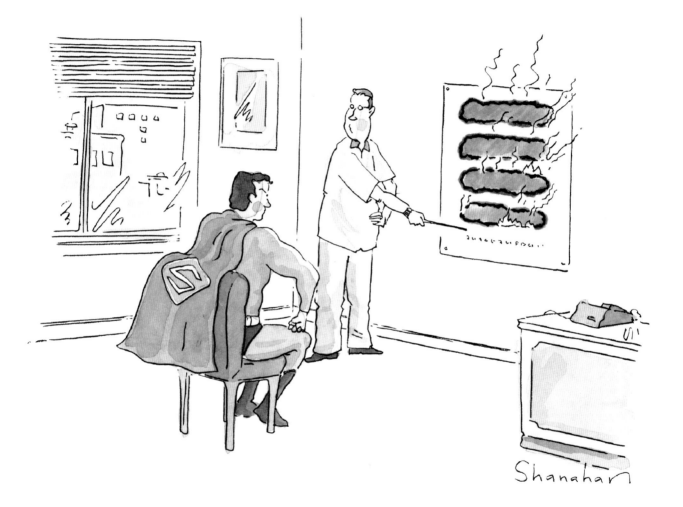

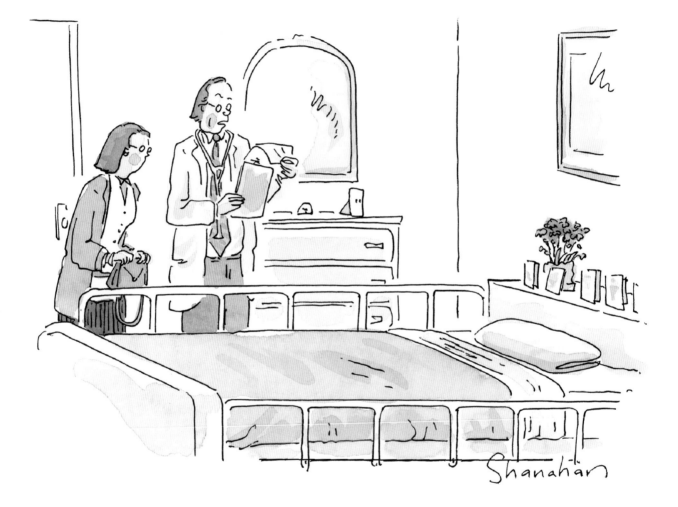

"Good news, Mrs. Bryant. I think we got it all."

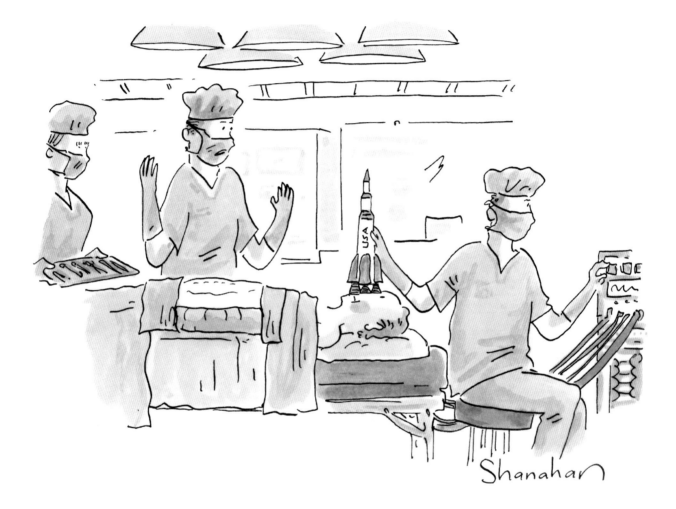

"Now start counting down from ten."

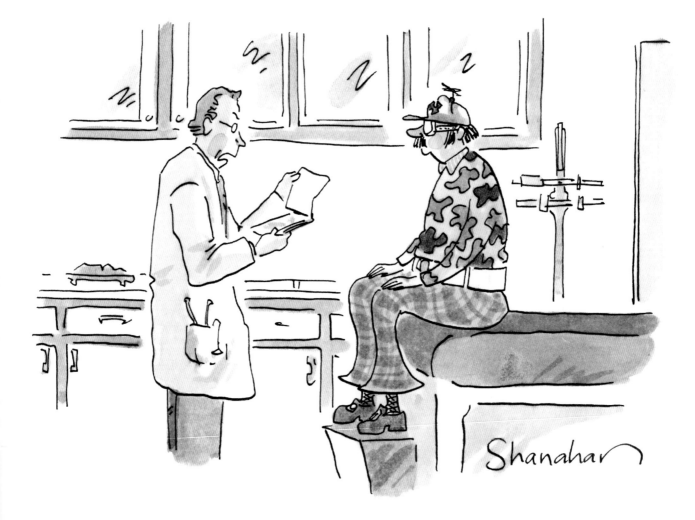

"The designer drugs aren't working."

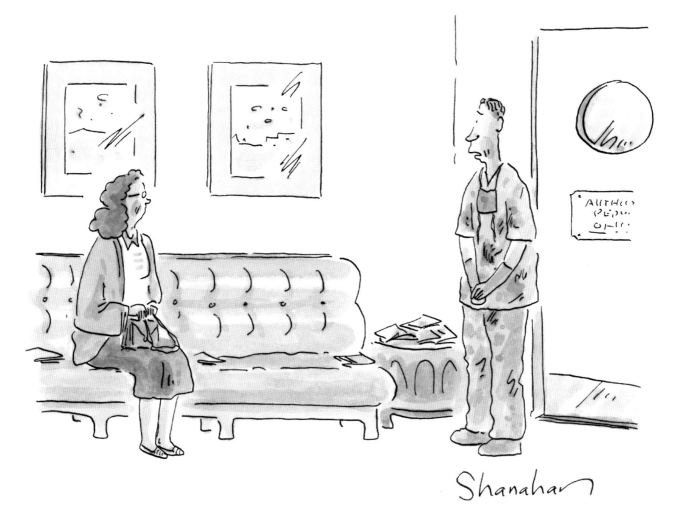

"My bad."

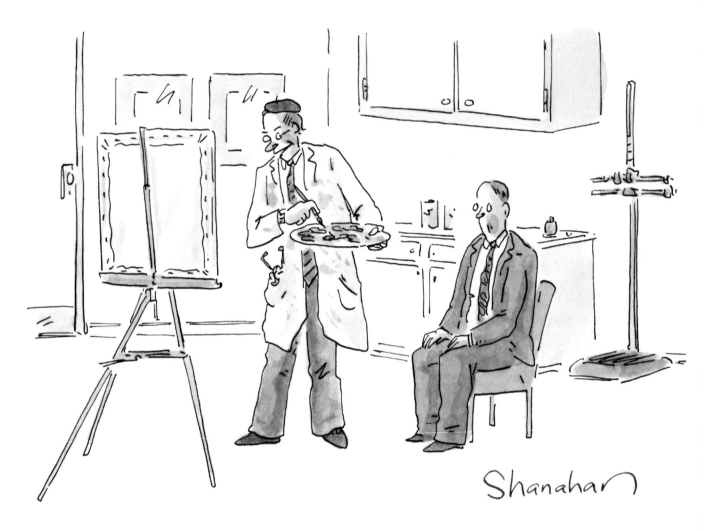

"O.K., Mr. Tuttle—describe your pain."

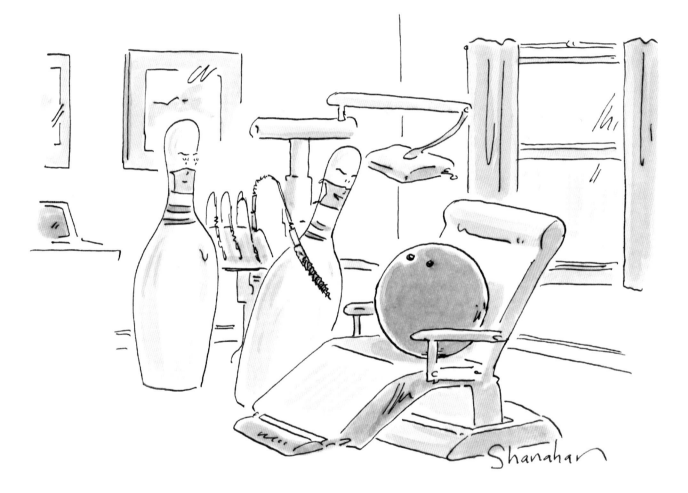

"You may experience a bit of discomfort."

Shanahan

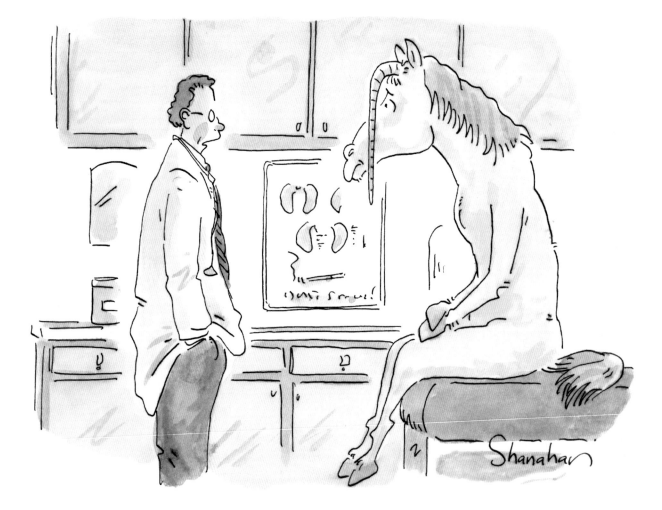

"*First, let me dispel all the myths.*"

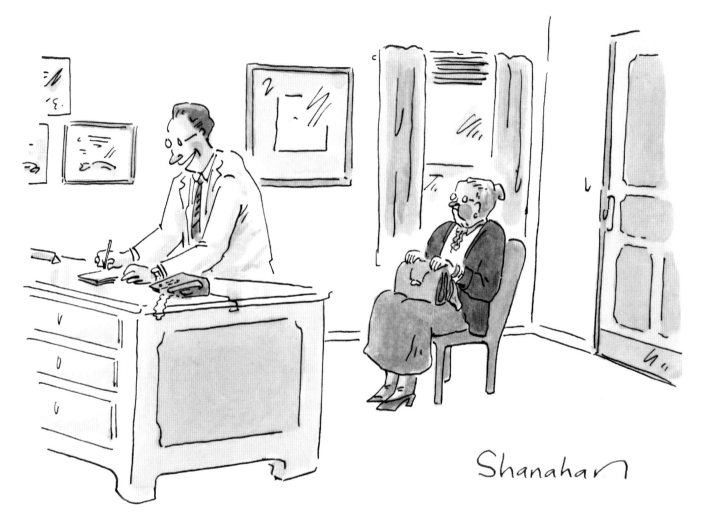

"*Your grandkids would* kill *for this prescription!*"

Shanahan

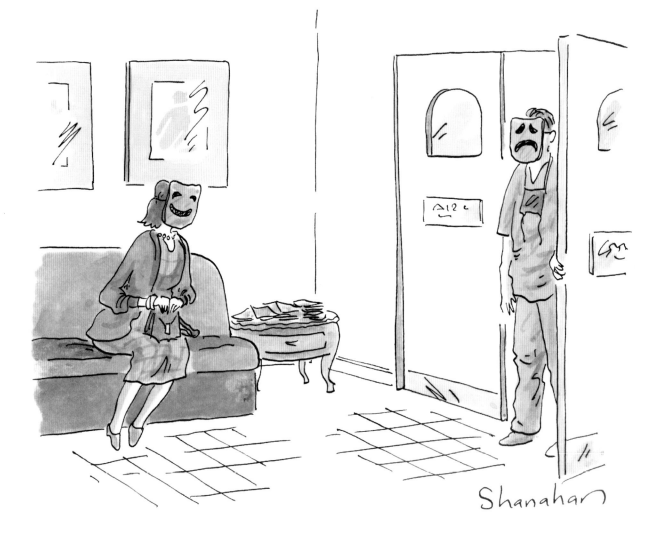

Shanahan

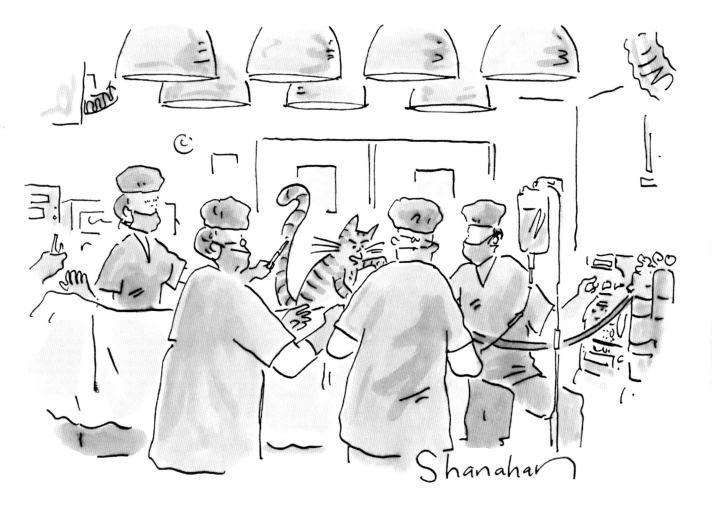

"O.K.—I've got the tongue."

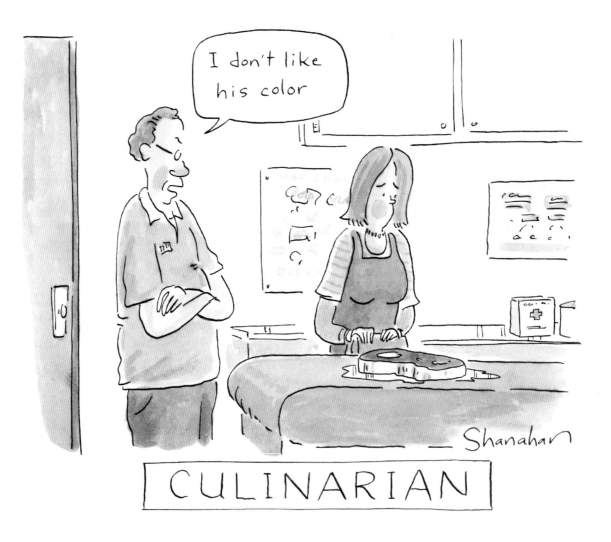

CULINARIAN

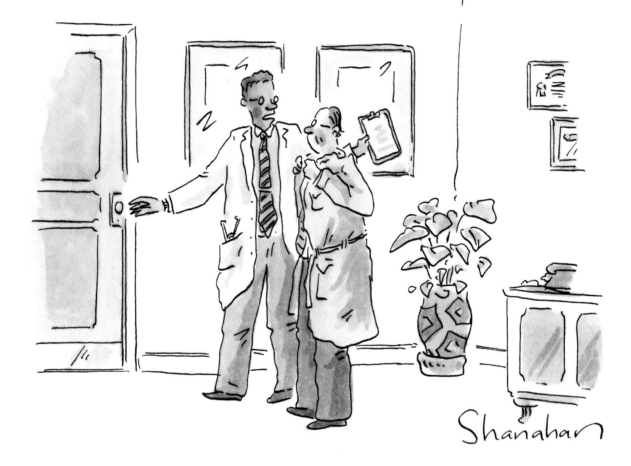

"*You're fit to stand trial, Mr. Douglas, so feel free to get out there and commit a crime.*"

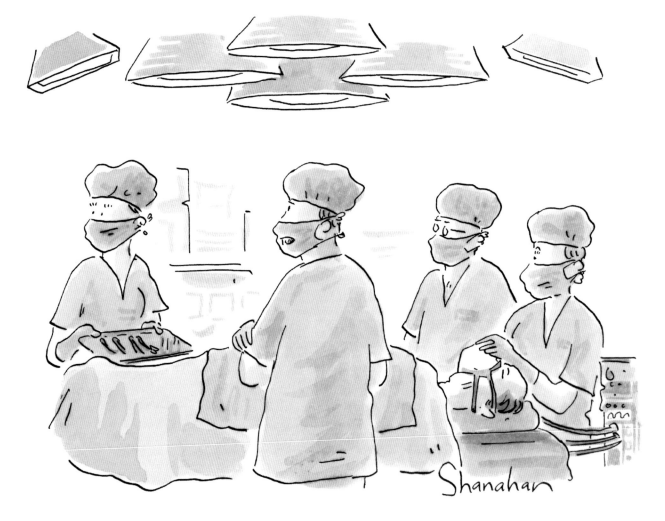

"Well, I'll be—he cut and ran."

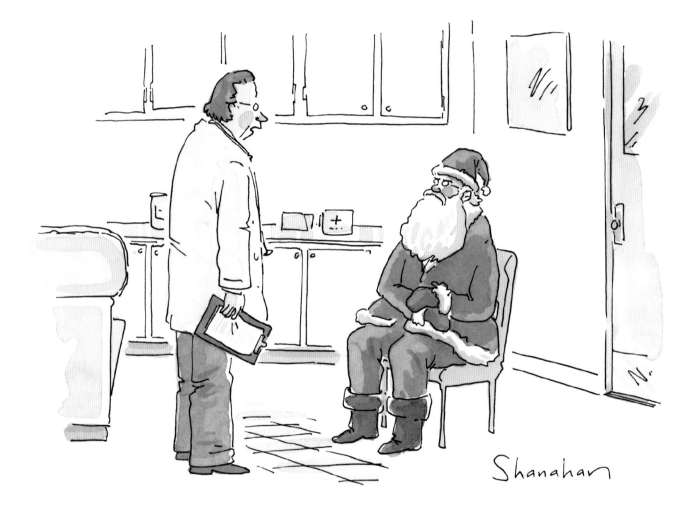

"It's Lyme disease again."

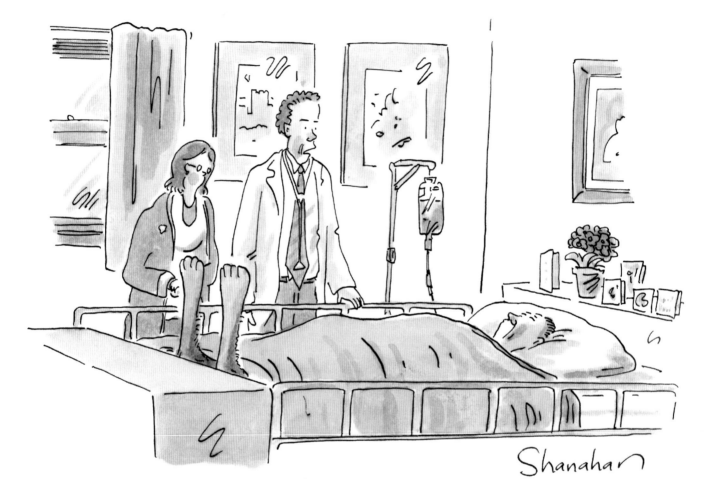

"He was very, very lucky."

Shanahan

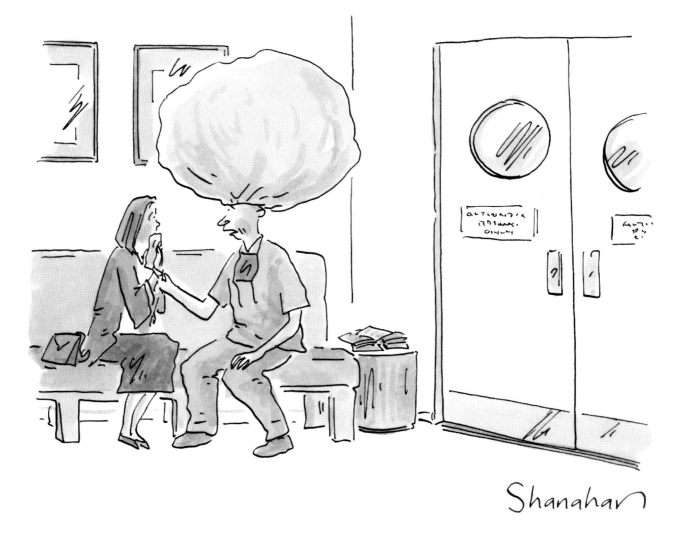

"Somehow a hair got into the incision."

Shanahan

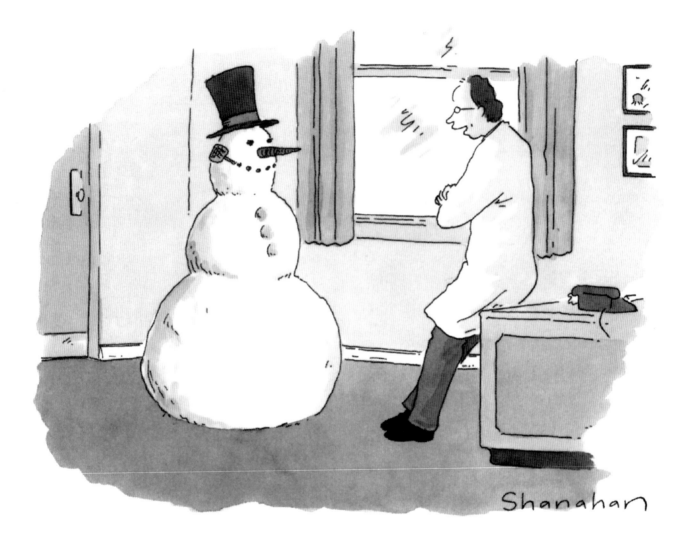

"Good news—those lumps were just coal."

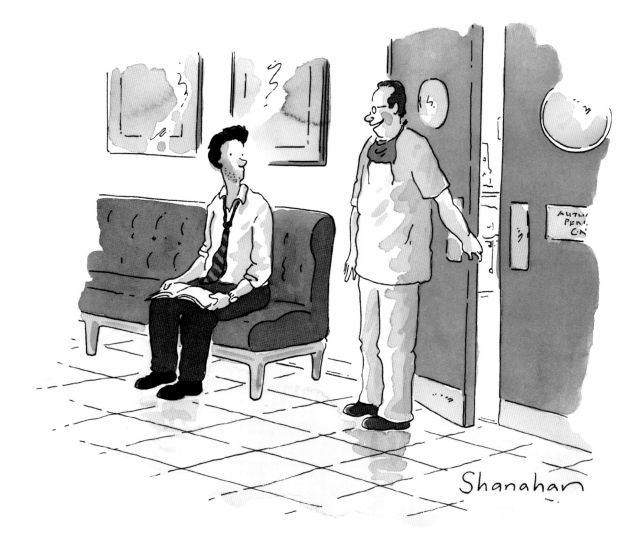

"*Congratulations! It's a Beanie Baby.*"

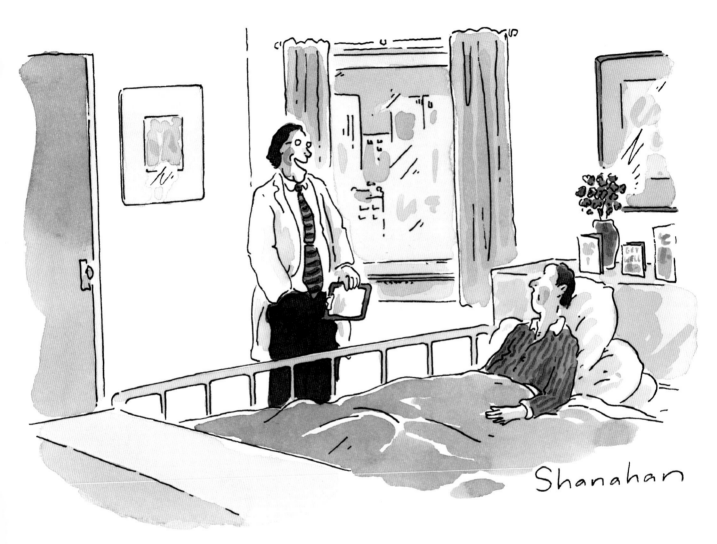

"And, in our continuing effort to minimize surgical costs, I'll be hitting you over the head and tearing you open with my bare hands."

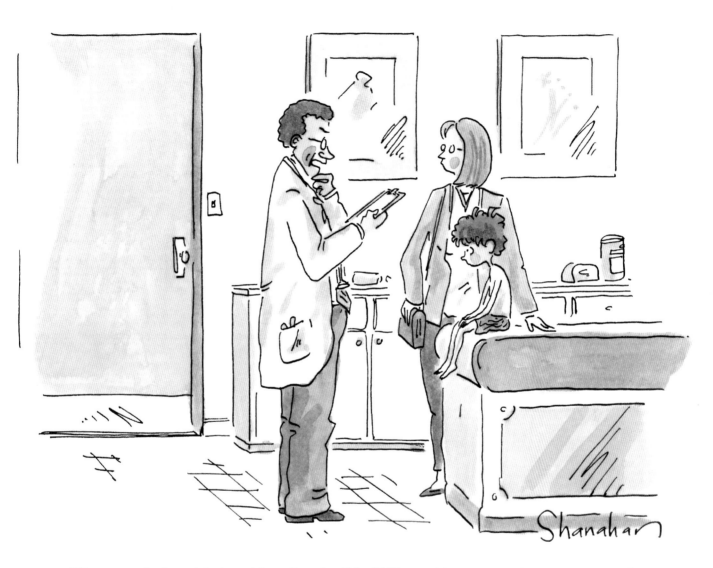

"He seems to be fine with the quirk quellers, but I'd still like to add an anomaly humbler to the mix."

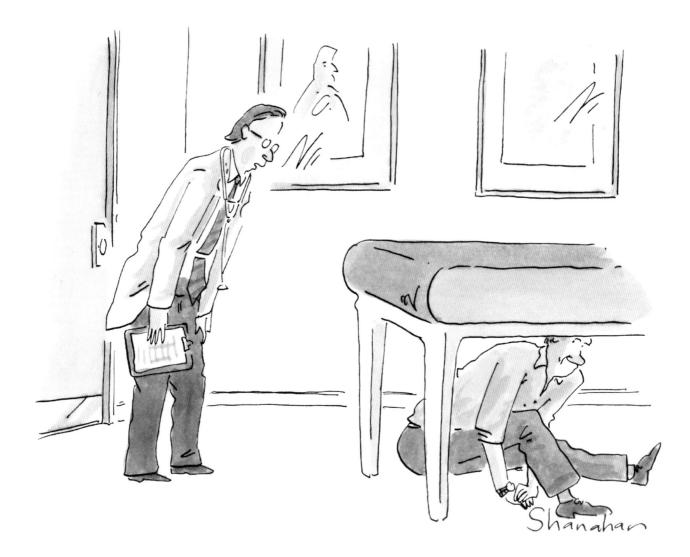

"So, Mr. Grossman, we've opted for the unexamined life?"

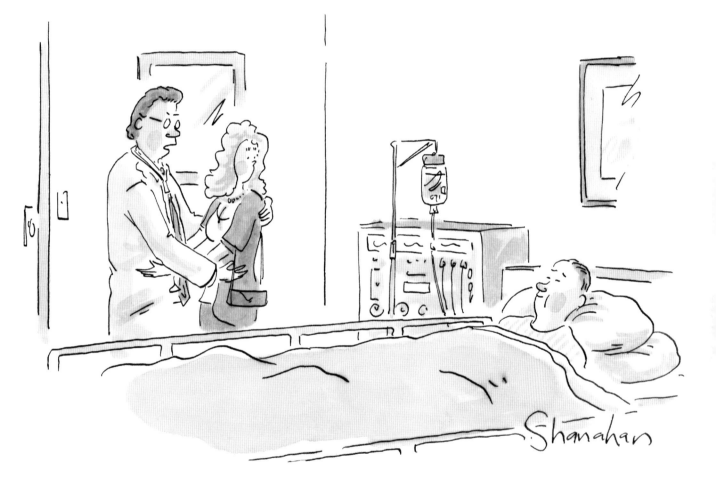

"*He seems benign, Mrs. Erlach, but I think it's best we had your husband removed.*"

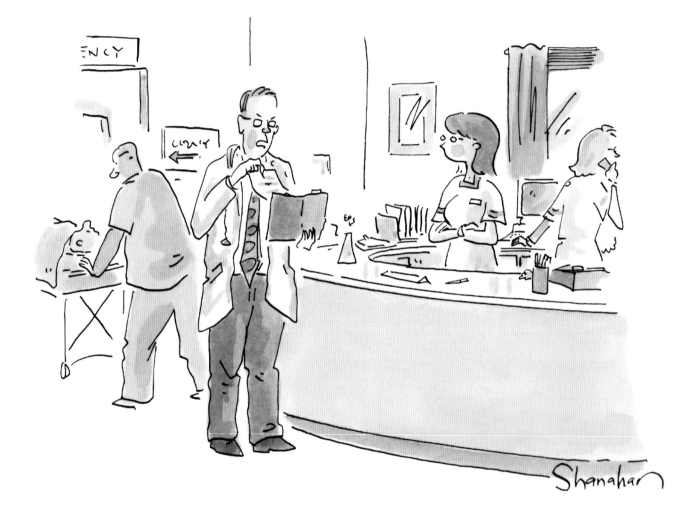

"He's not responding. Let's try some more aggressive billing."

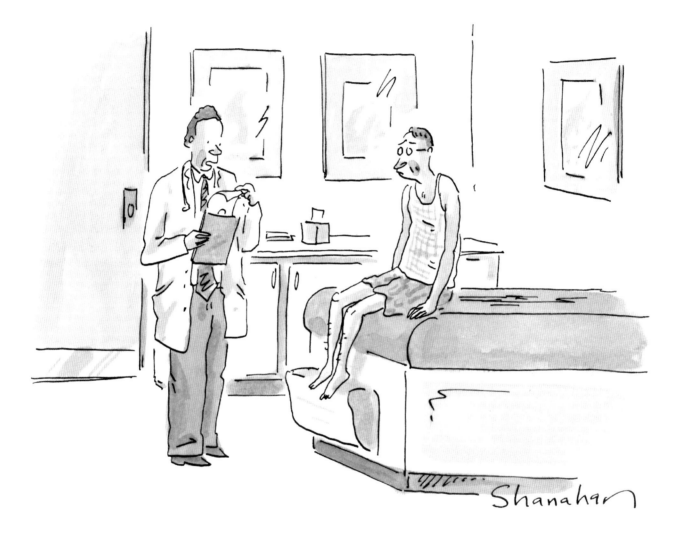

"And how long have you been feeling this way, Mr. Crapola?"

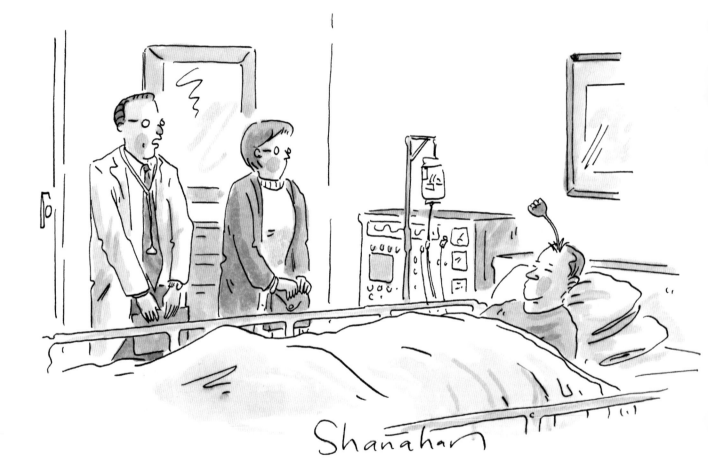

"It's inoperable and perennial."

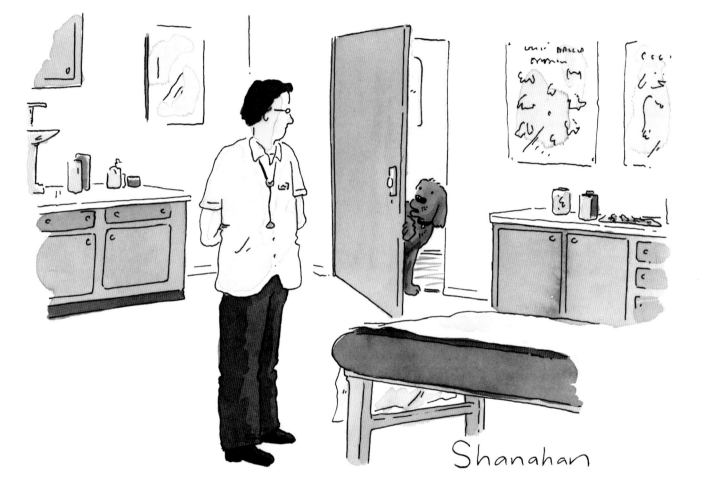

"I seem to have missed the cup."

Shanahan

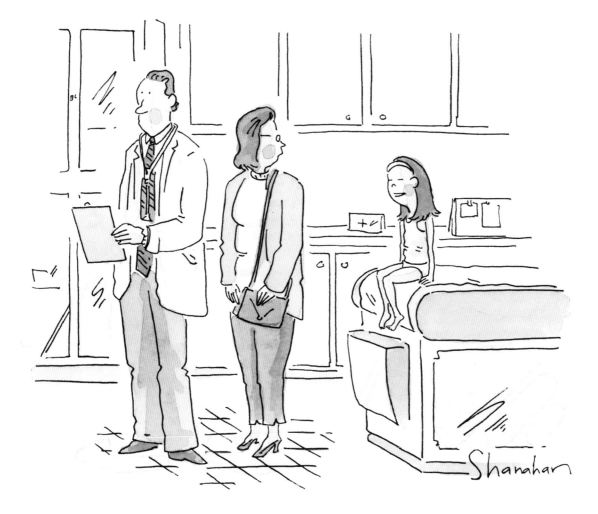

"*Bobby Linderman—now* there's *a doctor.*"

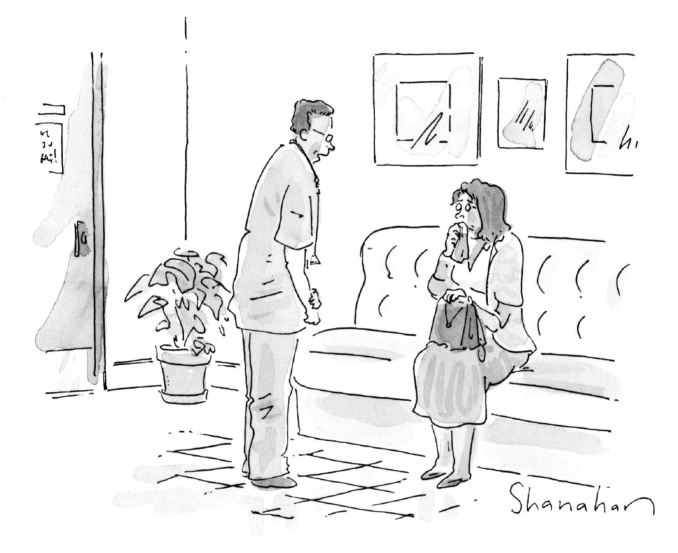

"If it's any consolation, toward the end he was as high as a kite."

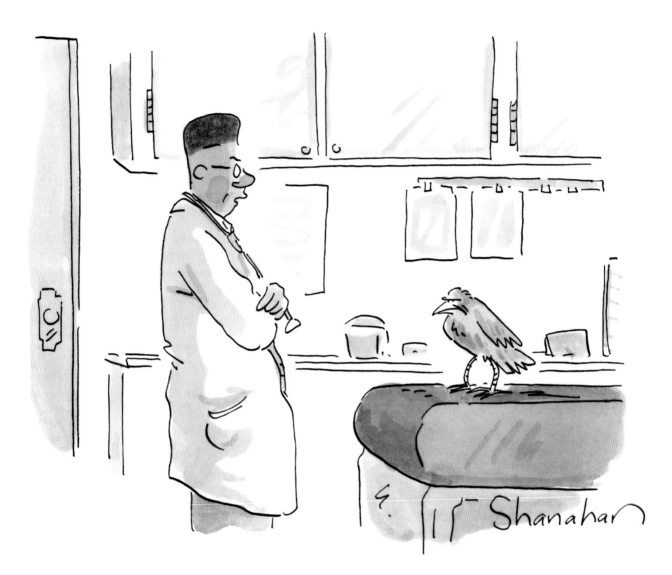

"It's time you had those dinosaur hips replaced."

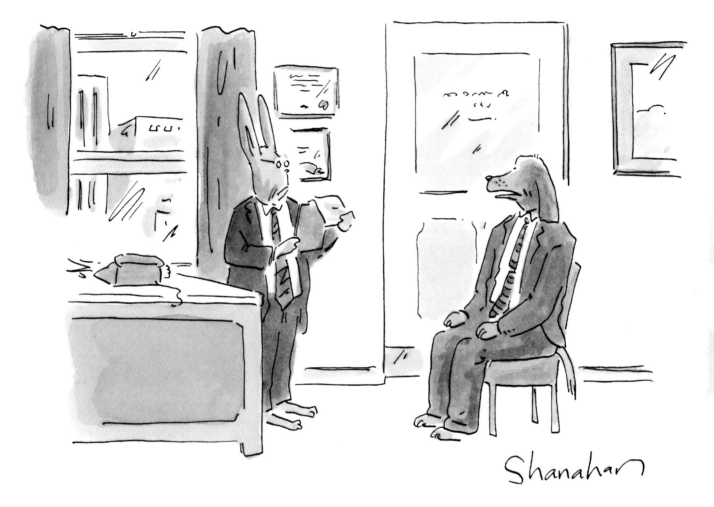

"My legs twitch in my sleep."

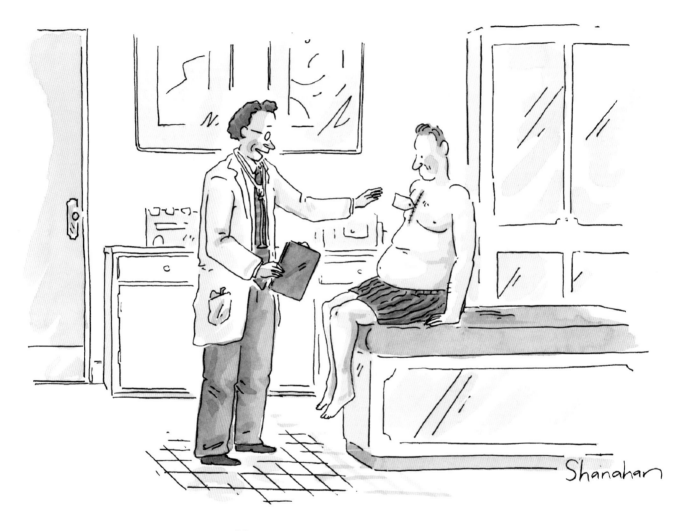

"Geez Louise—I left the price tag on."

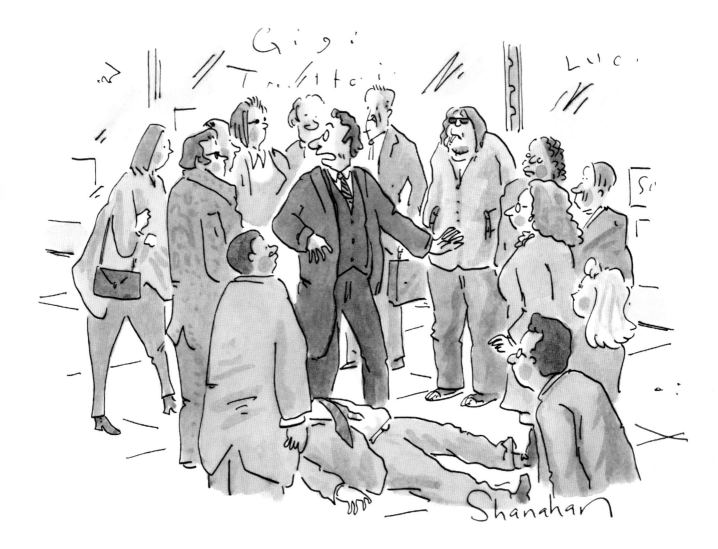

"Let me back out—that was my car alarm!"

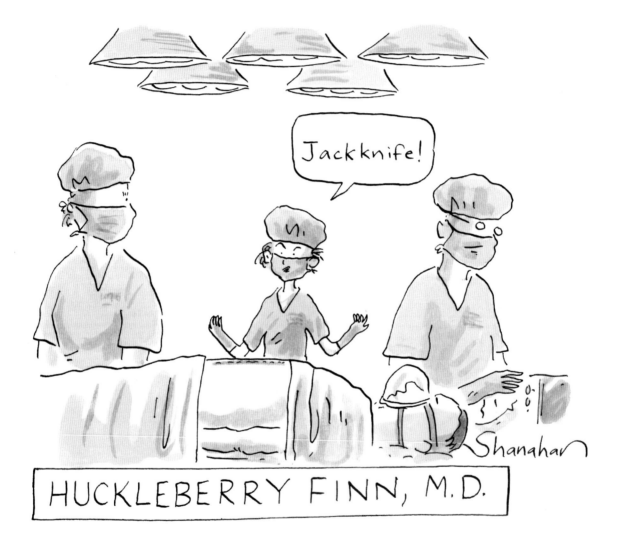

HUCKLEBERRY FINN, M.D.

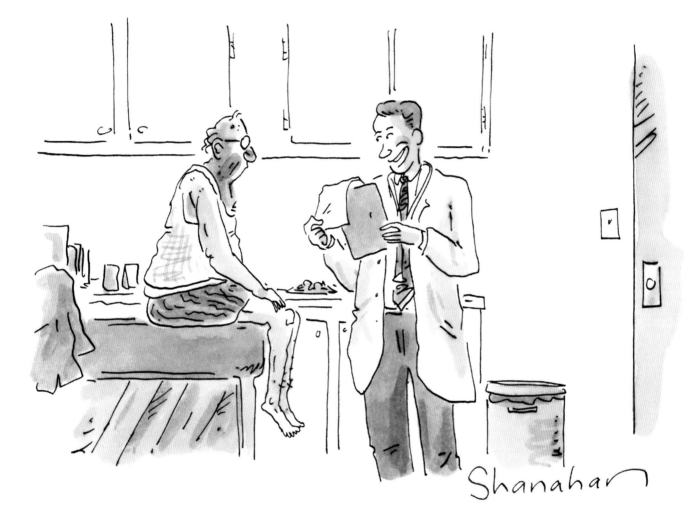

"*Nonsense, Mr. Turpin—you're as wealthy as an ox.*"

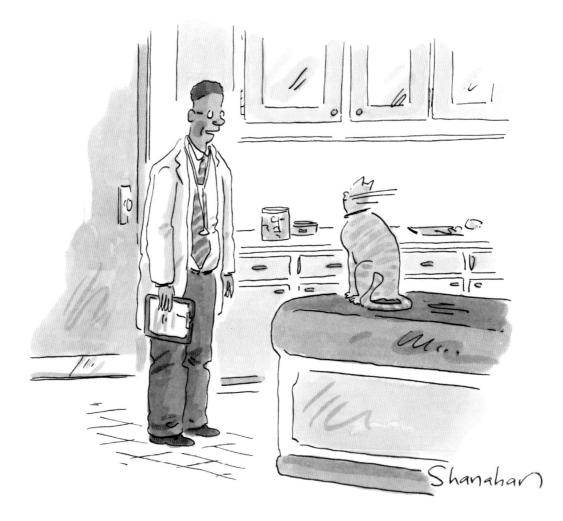

"Good news—it's not colon cancer, it's tinsel."

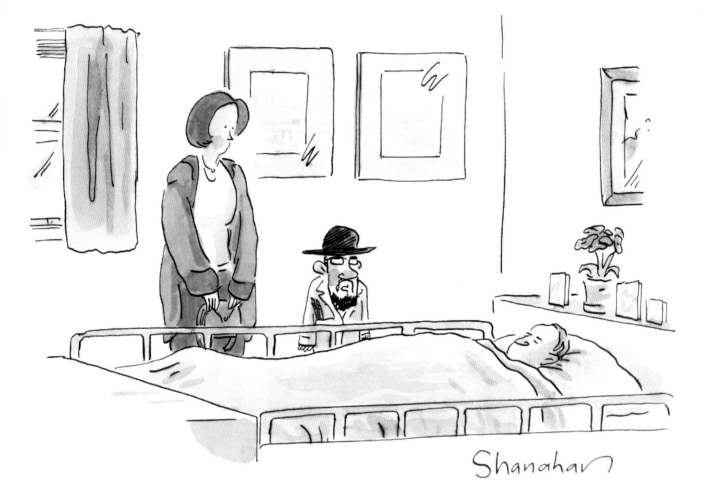

"*I don't like his color.*"

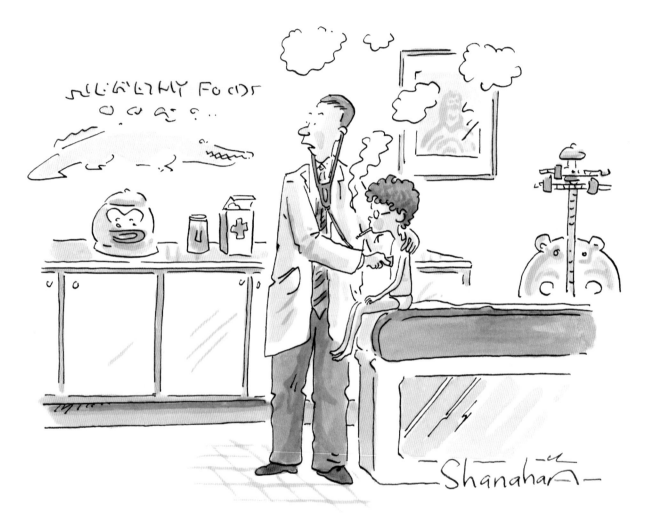

"One more deep drag."

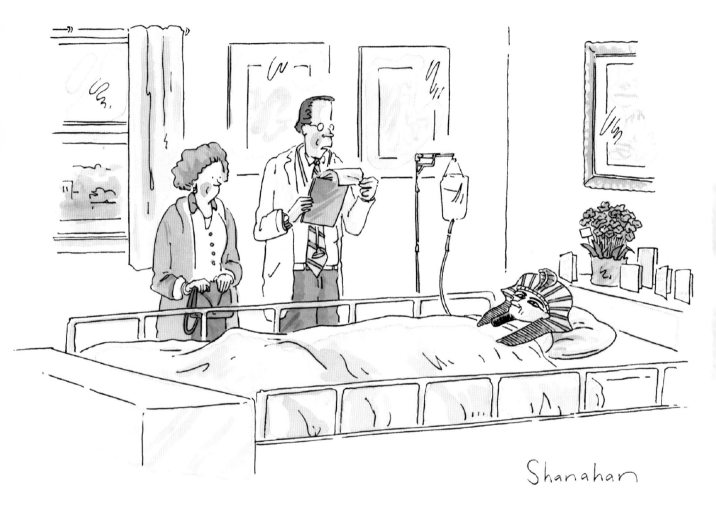

"We're pretty sure it's the West Nile virus."

Shanahan

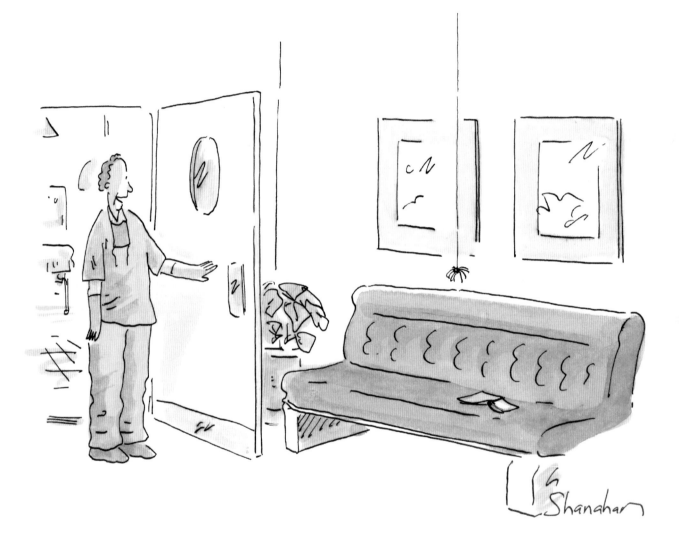

"Itsa bitsy."

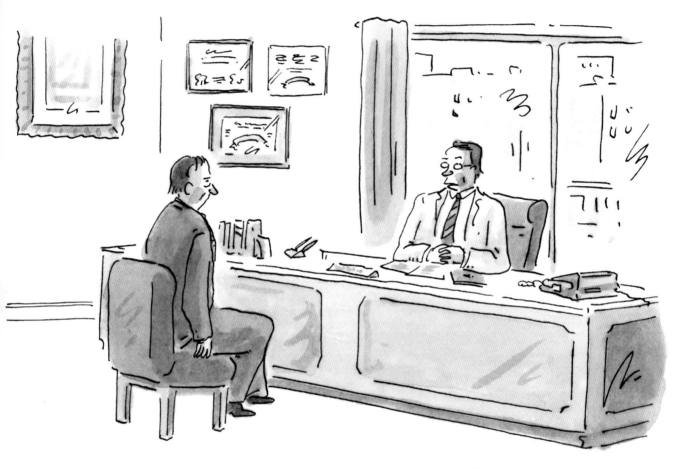

"You have Seasonal Affective Disorder, but your Attention Deficit Disorder will have you up and around in no time."

Shanahan

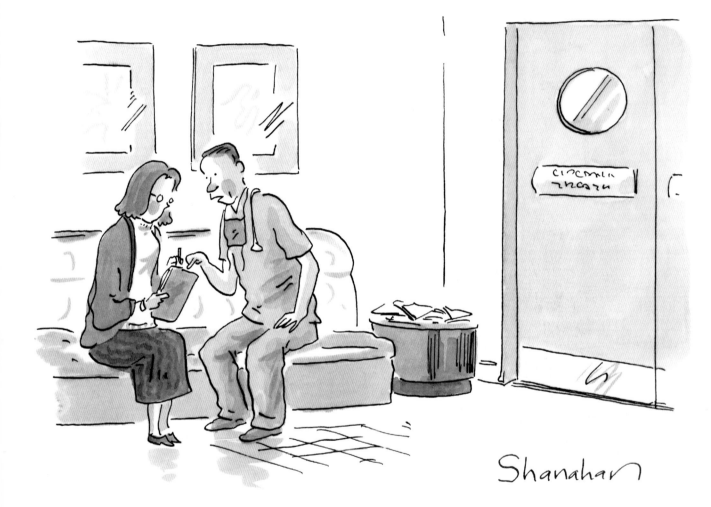

"And initial here if you'd like his balls in a sling."

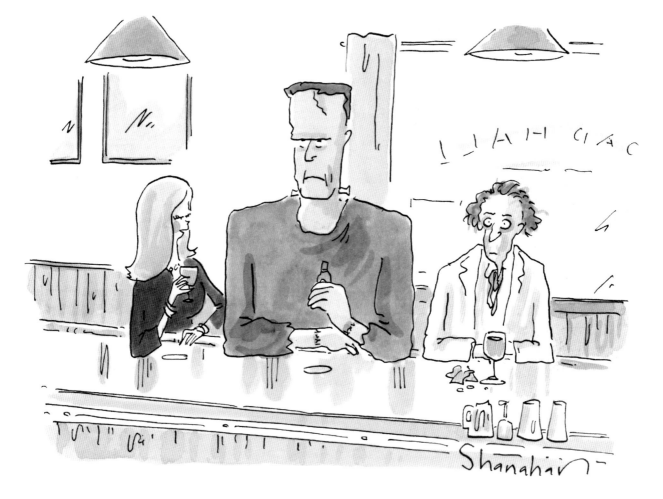

"So, your friend Victor's a doctor?"

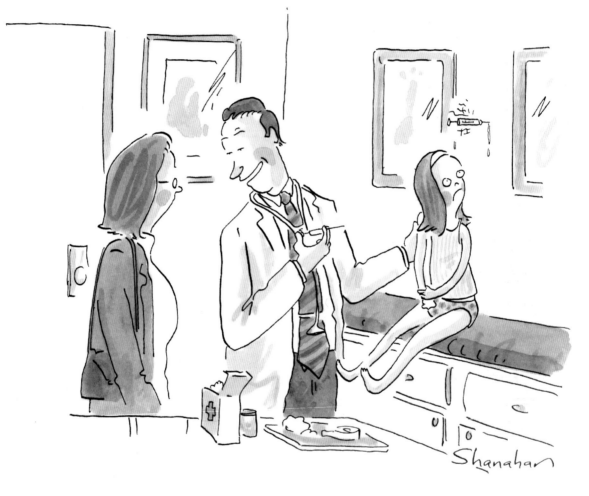

"The first one's just a warning."

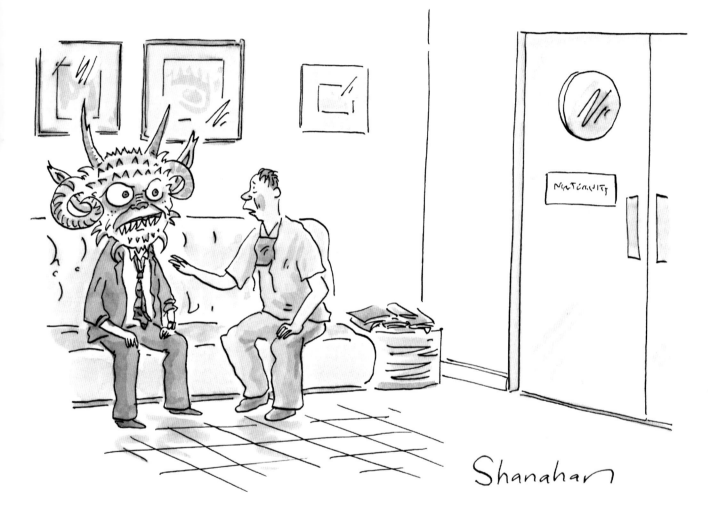

"It was a difficult delivery."

Shanahan

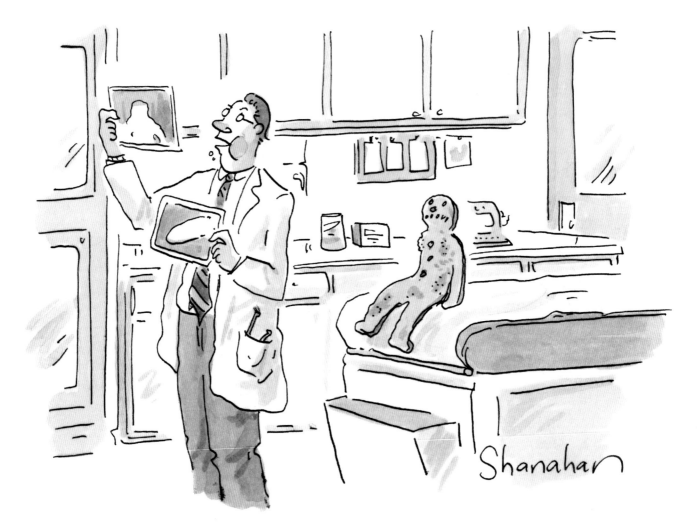

"Mmmm…yes…scrumptious—I think we got it all."

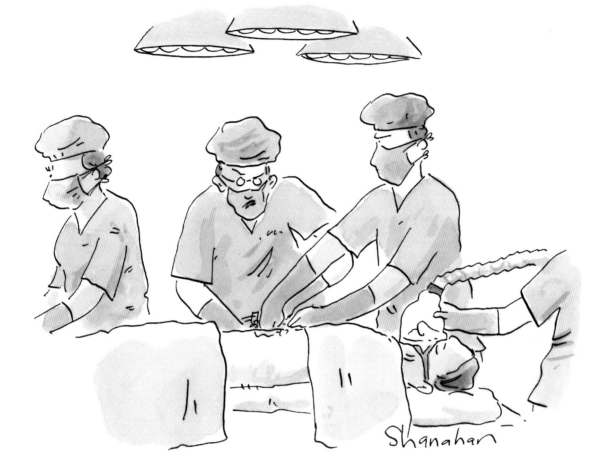

"And it'll stay clamped until you play my Usher CD."

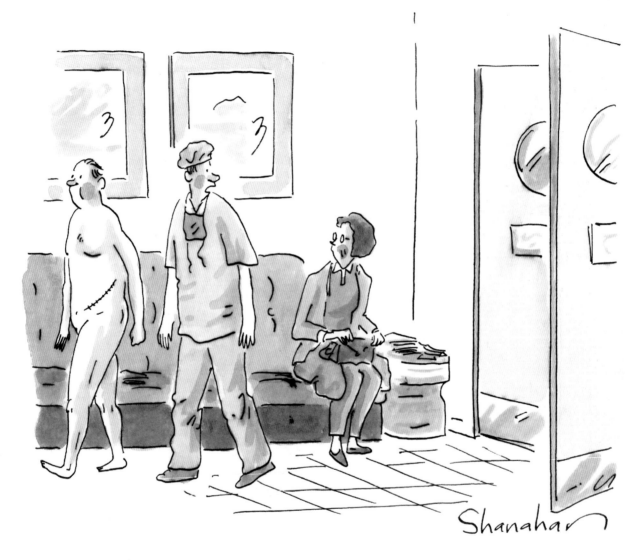

"I expect a speedy recovery."

Shanahan

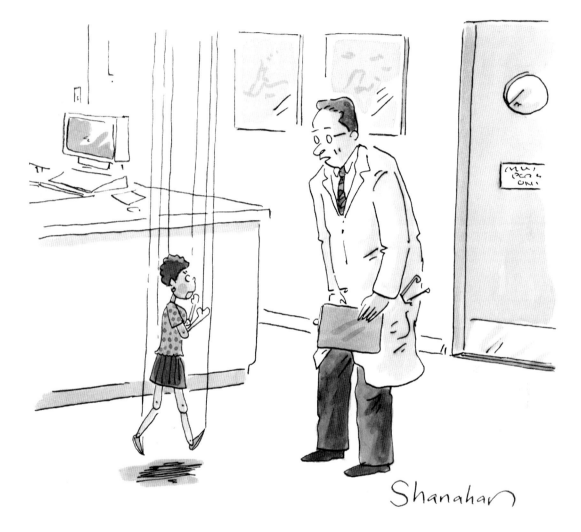

"I'm afraid it's his heartstring."

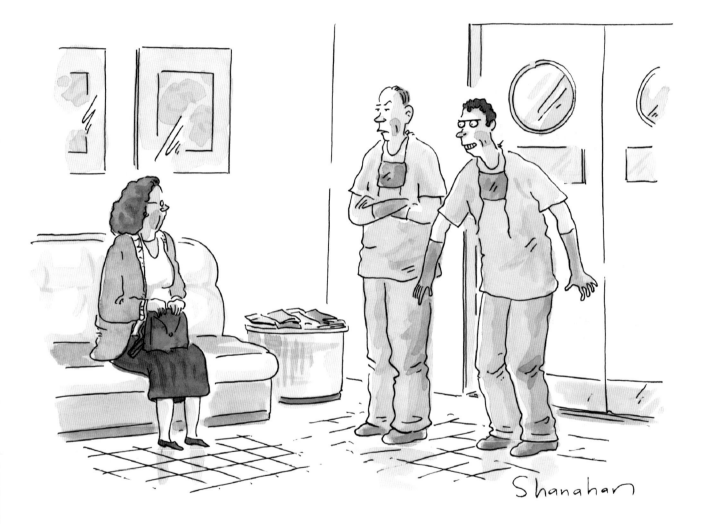

"What'll it be, Mrs. Waltham—stolid workmanship or nervy brilliance?"

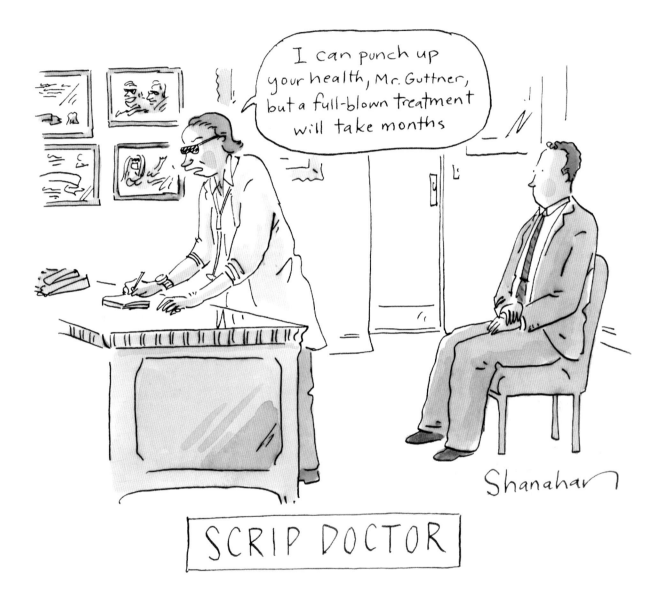

SCRIP DOCTOR

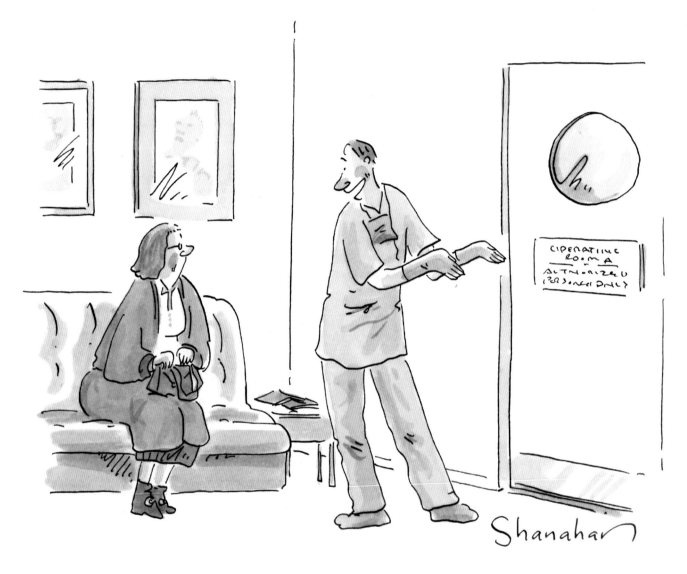

"*Thankfully, we were able to segue directly into an autopsy.*"

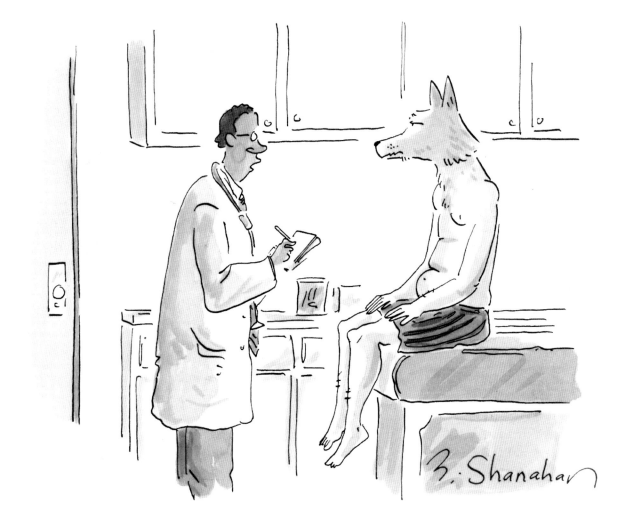

"*I'm referring you to an old gypsy woman.*"

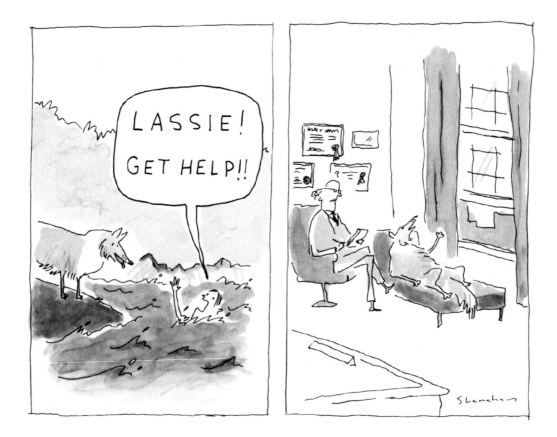

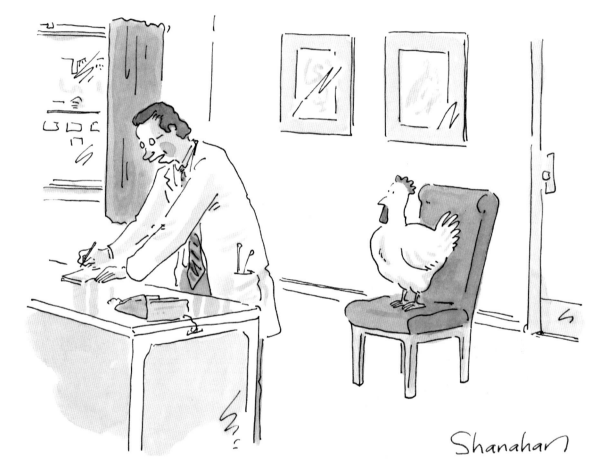

"But before you even think about going under the knife,
I'd like to recommend a good pluck and cook man."

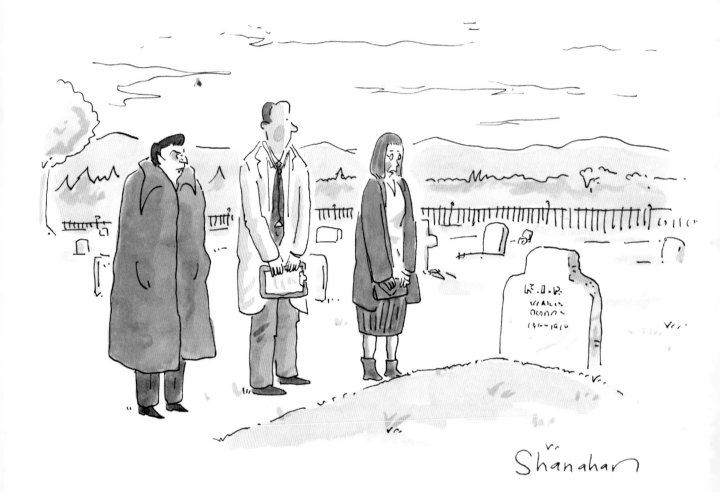

"Please—no more specialists."